Complete Guide to Juicing for a Healthy Life

Healthy Food Series #7
By Rod Stone

Copyright Notice

Disclaimer:

The information contained in this eBook is strictly for informational purposes. It is not intended as medical advice. Every possible effort has been made in preparing and researching this material. We make no warranties with respect to the accuracy, applicability of its contents or any omissions.

Table of Contents

Introduction...i

Benefits of Juicing 1

Juicing Versus Blending 5

Juicer Buying Guide..10

Best Fruits and Vegetables for Juicing 14

Herbs and Spices...24

Juicing Tips 41

Juicing for Specific Benefits 60

Juicing for Weight Loss 60

Juicing for Exercise...63

Juicing for Better Aging..82

Juicing for Cancer 95

Juicing for Skin Health 110

Plant Nutrition A to Z 119

Fruits 119

Vegetables 149

Recipes 185

Recipes for Exercise....................................185

Anti-Aging Juicing Recipes 190

Recipes for Healthy Skin 196

Green Juice Recipes.....................................201

20 Ways to Enjoy Raw Vegetables...............206

Conclusion 216

Introduction

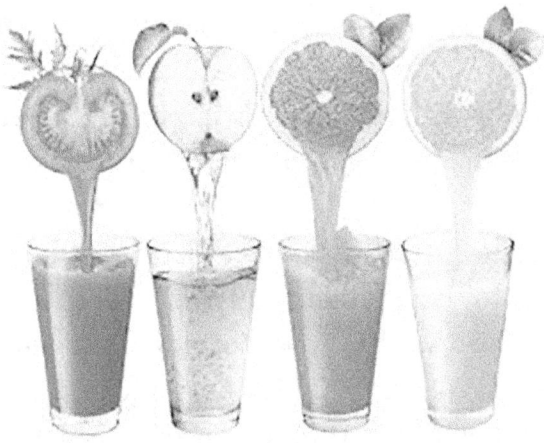

It's well documented that many of us need to increase our daily intake of fruit and vegetables. We are the champions of the world when it comes to getting enough carbs, protein, and fat, but we're sorely lacking when it comes to getting more micronutrients.

While the Centers for Disease Control recommend adults consume about 1 ½ to 2 cups of fruit and 2 to 3 cups of vegetables daily, an analysis of American diets between 2007 and 2010 found that 50% of the population ate less than 1 cup of fruit and less than 1 ½ cups of vegetables.

It has been shown that those who consume at least the recommended amounts of each are not only healthier but are also less likely to be overweight.

However, fruit and vegetables are where essential micronutrients are to be found and juicing is a great way to easily pack more of them into a well-balanced and healthy diet.

Juicing is a great way to get your body pumped and primed for a lengthy workout session. When you juice, you cram loads of essential nutrients into one glass that will power your workout and improve your results.

Besides the important health benefits, key plant nutrients give you energy so you perform at your best in your workouts and get the most out of your exercise efforts.

Juicing is a healthy practice that has allowed millions of people to boost their nutrition. Juicing fruits and vegetables provides you important antioxidants, which scavenge for oxygen free radicals that can damage cellular structures, including DNA. When DNA is damaged, it can result in mutations that lead to cancer.

Well-balanced nutrition from a variety of healthy whole foods helps support and maintain on going good health, and experts agree that nutrition plays a key role in preventing chronic and terminal illness.

Juicing is practiced by millions around the world and it is an easy and convenient way to get plant nutrition into the body to do its magic.

When juicing is done right, that is when the majority of your juice blends is comprised of vegetables and very low sugar fruit you can easily boost your nutritional intake thereby improving your health and lower your risks for cancer.

This is why we have decided to make this book the newest in our Healthy Food Series. We hope you will find it useful in helping to provide you with a healthy life.

Benefits of Juicing

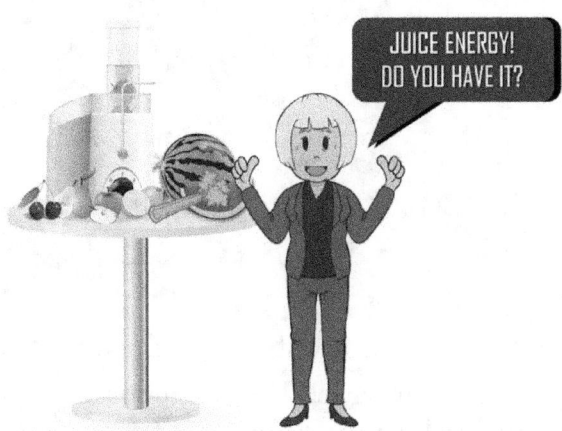

General Benefits of Juicing:

✓ Increased energy
✓ Improved immunity
✓ Stronger bones
✓ Improved hydration
✓ Better skin health and appearance
✓ Essential nutrients for general health and to fight chronic disease
✓ Weight loss
✓ Improve the aging process

Juice Nutrition

Juicing is a very convenient and easy way to consume healthier plant foods and the essential nutrients they provide.

Nutrients Exclusive to Vegetables and Fruits

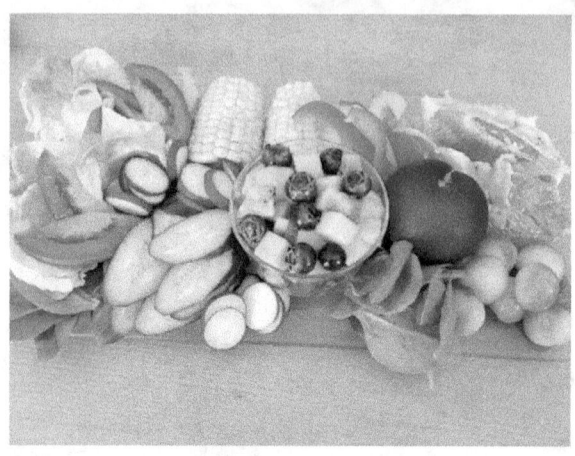

There are micronutrients in produce that you cannot get from any other food. This includes key antioxidants that fight free radicals and protect cells in the body.

Potassium

Potassium promotes proper fluid balance and supports muscle and nerve function. Fresh vegetables are key sources of potassium, including squash, artichokes, carrots, and broccoli.

Vitamin A

Vitamin A supports skin and vision health and also promotes immune system health. Yellow, orange, and dark leafy greens are the best sources, including cell peppers, kale, broccoli, and carrots.

Vitamin C

Vitamin C is a well-rounded antioxidant that enhances the absorption of iron, speeds wound healing and supports immune system health. Citrus fruits, like oranges, lemons, and grapefruits along with broccoli, tomatoes, and green pepper are some of the best sources.

Magnesium

Magnesium supports healthy bones and plays a key role in more than three hundred enzymes in the body.

Folate

Folate is a B-vitamin that plays a key role in the synthesis of red blood cells. Folate is a big part of prenatal vitamins as it prevents birth defects in the growing fetus. Broccoli, tomato juice, and asparagus are your best plant sources of folate.

Phytonutrients

According to the National Cancer Institute, phytonutrients may play a key role in preventing cancer and lowering risks for various health problems. Phytonutrients are active compounds found in plants that protect the plant from pests and other environmental hazards and they do the same for humans.

Three types of phytonutrients

- Organo-sulfurs – mainly found in garlic compounds
- Terpenoids – mainly found in citrus fruits
- Flavonoids - Flavonoids give fruits and vegetables their bright colors, like the red tomato and the purple grape, and the blue blueberry. This group includes the anthocyanins found in blueberries and the quercetin in onions.
- Isoflavonoids and lignans: Broccoli and curly kale are rich sources of lignans, along with cabbage, Brussels sprouts, carrots, and green peppers

Phytochemicals in Fruit

Anthocyanidins found in raspberries, blueberries, blackberries and purple and red grapes help protect from the damaging effects of oxidation.

Phytochemicals in Vegetables - Glucosinolates

According to the National Cancer Institute, cruciferous vegetables, which are part of the brassica family of vegetables, including turnips, rutabaga, watercress, broccoli, kale, cabbage, and bok choy appear to have significant cancer-preventive properties.

cabbage, and bok choy appear to have significant cancer-preventive properties.

Various studies show these vegetables to prevent cancer in different ways:

- Protect cells from DNA damage
- Ability to inactivate carcinogens
- Hold antiviral, anti-inflammatory and antibacterial properties
- Induce apoptosis or cell death
- Hinder tumor blood vessel formation and migration, which is required for metastasis

Juicing Versus Blending

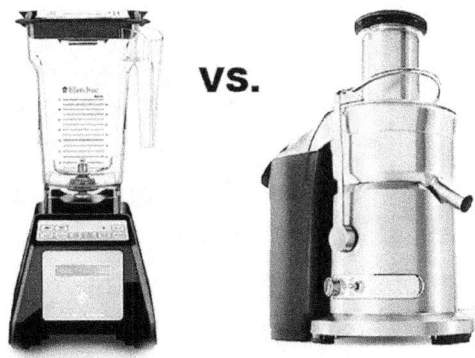

A common question that is often asked is what is better? Juicing or blending?

People often ask whether juicing offers more health benefits, or whether blending is the way to go. First of all, let's take a look at the differences between the two.

When you juice fruits and vegetables, you're essentially extracting the water and the nutrients and leaving the pulp behind. Conversely, blenders pulverize the entire fruit and vegetable and instead of making juice, you get what is called a smoothie.

There are many health benefits to both juicing and blending, thanks to all the vitamins, phytonutrients and minerals, you're getting everything you need for a healthier you.

Whether you're looking to refuel after a workout, or just need a quick and healthy meal you can enjoy on the run, blending and juicing let you pack several servings of fruits and veggies into one glass.

Blend for More Fiber

The main difference is that the pulp contains insoluble fiber, which is missing from the juice because the pulp is removed.

Most people need more fiber in their diet. The average American downs only 14 grams of fiber per day, which is just over half the daily need for women and one-third of what men require. And these numbers are still considered low by many people. They show that the hunter gathers of years ago would have between 60-150 grams per day.

Choosing fiber-free juice over fiber-filled smoothies also means your beverage won't be as satisfying as it could be. Fiber naturally regulates your blood sugar levels and absorbs water in your digestive tract, which means you feel fuller longer. If you opt for juice over a smoothie, the lack of fiber combined with the blood sugar spike might leave you ravenous in an hour or two.

Fiber is essential for long-term health, too. It absorbs cholesterol in your digestive tract and flushes it out of your body, which is helpful for reducing risk factors for heart disease. Meals high in fiber also keep your digestive system moving, preventing constipation.

Insoluble Fiber

Insoluble fiber is mainly found in whole wheat, brown rice and in the seeds and skins of fruit. It digests slowly and so results in a slower and more sustained release of nutrients.

Health Benefits of Insoluble Fiber:
- Supports weight loss as it keeps you full longer so you eat less without being hungry

- Supports healthy digestion, and prevents bowel problems
- People often drink a smoothie before a workout to give them a slow and sustained energy drip because the insoluble fiber digests slower than the soluble fiber found in juices

Soluble Fiber

While there is no insoluble fiber in juice, you are still getting a lot of soluble fiber. Soluble fiber attracts water and turns to gel during the digestive process, and causes slower digestion, it is found in apples, blueberries, other fruits and vegetables, beans, nuts, seeds and oat bran, and it is the main ingredient in psyllium fiber supplements.

Soluble fiber absorbs quickly and easily, allowing you to get 100% of key vitamins, minerals, and antioxidants from juiced fruits and vegetables.

Health Benefits of Soluble Fiber

- Helps keep cholesterol levels healthy and protects the heart.
- Bulks up the stool to support healthy digestion and prevent common ailments, such as diarrhea and constipation and diarrhea. This is why fiber supplements are made mostly from soluble fiber.
- Maintains healthy blood sugar levels to avoid blood sugar spikes that pose a risk for type 2 diabetes and can help those already diagnosed to manage the condition.
- Soluble fiber supports weight loss as it can keep you full longer, while keeping your calorie counts

down, especially when its source is fruits and vegetables.

- Older people and those with digestive disorders can benefit from juicing and eliminate the hard to digest insoluble fiber found in juiced or whole fruits and vegetables.

Which Is Better: Juicing or Blending?

The answer is both are great! But fiber is so important I recommend blending. But if you cannot afford a powerful blender than stay with juicing.

- ✓ Juicing vegetables allows you to get a plethora of key nutrients without the bulk of the insoluble fiber for pure liquid nutrition.
- ✓ Blending and juicing together allows you to make a variety of tasty blends, for example, strawberries don't juice very well, but kale, and spinach does. Therefore, you make your vegetable juice, and then stir in the blended strawberries, and you get the best of both worlds, delicious taste and complete nutrition.
- ✓ Blending is ideal for the soft produce that cannot be juiced, like avocados, and bananas.
- ✓ Blending also allows you to get the benefits of the entire fruit, as the fiber content prevents the blood sugar spikes that are seen with high sugar fruit juices.
- ✓ If you want to boost the nutritional value of your diet, juicing gives you a straight shot of nutrition any time of the day. You don't have to spend all day deciding what fruit or vegetable to eat next - you can get all your nutrients in one go. Excellent!

✓ Juicing allows for an easy way to drink your nutrition, instead of having to chew on a giant plate of vegetables or drinking a thick smoothie. Juicing gives you more choices, due to the great variety of judicable fruits and vegetables.

Sound nutrition is so important, but so many of us just don't get enough. We are great at getting our macronutrients (protein, carbs, and fat) but we're not so great when it comes to getting enough micronutrients. Juicing and blending is a great way to boost our intake of micronutrients and improve our diets.

The great thing about juices and smoothies is that they allow you to get more fruit and vegetables than you otherwise would.

After all, you can only chew so much kale each day, or peel so many apples.

You get exhausted doing it. You forget to do it.

Juicing and blending makes everything so much easier and so portable.

Blend to Reduce Food Waste

Fruits and veggies are the most wasted food, according to an Environmental Protection Agency report, accounting for almost half of the total food waste in America in 2010.

Opting to blend ensures you keep all the goodness of the produce in your smoothie, virtually eliminating waste. When you juice, you increase food waste as you end up throwing out the pulp. And because you can't separate all the juice from the pulp, you're also wasting some fresh, nutrient-rich juice.

Juicer Buying Guide

There are two main types of juicers:
- Centrifugal juicer (fast juicers)
- Masticating juicer (slow juicers)

Centrifugal Juicers

Centrifugal or fast juicers are the most popular type of juicer. Why do people love centrifugal juicers? Because they're fast! It's their biggest selling point. If you're looking to make a juice fast, then centrifugal juicers are a good option. They speed up the process, and they clean easy too.

In addition, you get a LOT of juice from your fruit and vegetables, especially if you've invested in a good one.

Fast juicers work by using a centrifugal force that draws out the produce's juicy goodness. The spinning motion much like that of a washing machine separates the juice from the pulp.

The produce is forced down a feed tube (you can just dump whole fruits in there, no need for chopping) before they meet a serrated cutting blade that spins at around 12,000 RPM. The shredded pulp goes into a basket, while the juice goes into a separate container.

Pros
- They juice fast so they are ideal for busy people
- Space saving smaller models
- Do not require the pre-cutting of produce so they save time on prep work
- Work great with hard vegetables, like cucumbers

Cons

- Not the best choice for leafy greens as they will extract less juice than masticating juicers
- Lower juice yield
- Oxidization
- Very noisy models

Masticating Juicers

Masticating or slow juicers do not shred produce with blades, but instead use a slow rotating auger to crush produce against a stainless steel mesh screen at only 80 to 100 rpm, creating no oxidation.

With slow juicers, you get a higher yield and slow juicers are particularly good at making green juices because they get the best nutrients out of kale, spinach and so on.

Pros

- Ideal for leafy greens and can juice wheatgrass
- High juice yield
- No oxidation
- Many models can also make nut butters, juice wheatgrass and even make sorbet

Cons

- More prep work due to a smaller feed chute
- Costlier than centrifugal models
- Take more time to extract juice, so slower than centrifugal juicers
- Large and bulky so will need more counter space

- Leaves more pulp in the juice, so may require a strainer (depending on your needs, this may be a pro)

Juicer Shopping Considerations
Juicers Do Not Come Cheap

Juicers are not cheap, so when you consider your purchase, think about this, is juicing just going to be a luxury in your life, or is it going to become a crucial, even necessary part of your new lifestyle? Will you juice ever day or every month?

If juicing is going to be a fundamental part of your life, then it is smart to invest in the best juicer you can afford. If, however, you're only going to be juicing every now and then, then consider a less expensive model that will do the job.

Easy to Use and Clean

This maybe one of your most important considerations because if you have a busy life, spending 20 minutes chopping and prepping ingredients and another 15 minutes on cleaning will be a hassle. In this case, choose a juicer with a big feed chute, the bigger, and the better, as this will require little or no chopping of produce.

There Are Powerful Juicers ... And There Are REALLY Powerful Juicers

There are the really colossal juicers and there are smaller juicers. The bigger models will be very big and powerful, and may be not ideal for novices or even younger family members like teenagers.

If you're just starting out in juicing, consider this in your shopping. If you have a large household, you may want a much larger model that can make more juice for lots of people, versus a one or two-person household where a smaller model is idea.

You should also bear in mind that the bigger the juicer is, the harder it's going to be to clean.

Best Fruits and Vegetables

for Juicing

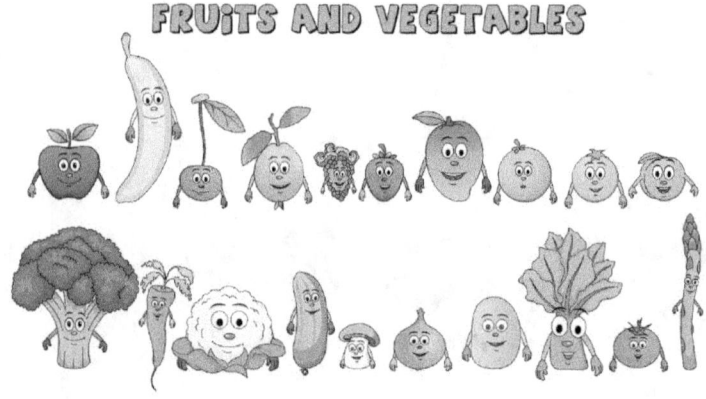

Here are some of the top fruits and vegetables to put in your juicer, as they are full of quality nutrients and are extremely supportive of good health. Please note that this list is by no means exhaustive and really most all fruits and vegetables can be juiced, though not all will yield the same amount of juice. Whichever you choose, keep in mind that juicing is pretty much a nutrient express train that zooms through your body rapidly. Think of it like a delivery driver who is trying to make record time!

Apples

Rich in antioxidants that fight the nasty toxins that swim around our bloodstream, apples give your health a boost in numerous ways. They can make your teeth whiter, help you to guard against Alzheimer's, prevent certain cancers, and reduce your risk of diabetes and lower cholesterol.

They're an amazing fruit that should really be an essential ingredient in your juices. They are also on the list of the lower sugar content fruit, and especially the green varieties, like Granny Smiths.

Broccoli

Broccoli is considered by kids everywhere and likely some adults to be a really boring vegetable, but broccoli is really supportive of human health and nutrition.

Athletes, bodybuilders, and health nuts include this cruciferous vegetable in their diet to prevent certain cancers, reduce cholesterol, strengthen bones, and help keep their bodies nice and toned. It is high in vitamin K and vitamin E, an antioxidant that protects cells from free radicals, as well as B vitamins AND vitamin C that boosts immunity.

Broccoli juices great and blends well with apples, pears, and even berries.

Berries

Berries are probably the easiest, smallest fruit you will ever juice. They're super convenient, super tasty, and they're absolutely crammed with goodness that contributes to a healthier you.

Berries are rich in essential antioxidants to protect cells from free radical damage and they are low in sugar. Perhaps you prefer blackberries today and tomorrow you want to make a strawberry-based juice. Or how about blueberries or raspberries instead? The choice is yours.

Berries do not always juice as well as other fruit, however you can blend them and stir into your vegetable juices, and this also helps to retain their insoluble fiber. Raspberries and blackberries are your lowest sugar options, and blueberries and strawberries have a low to medium sugar content.

Cabbage

Cabbage is another great base juice as it is 95% water. If you are like most people, you probably don't like eating cabbage whole. It's big, it's chewy, and it just doesn't go down too well. When you juice it, though, it's pretty amazing.

You can actually juice cabbage on its own, though its flavor is much enhanced by apples or carrots. Cabbage juice helps you to lose weight by purifying your intestine so that disposing of waste becomes so much easier. It can also protect you from certain cancers, ward off cataracts, and strengthen your immune system.

Carrots

Carrots add some color to your juice, but there is much more to them as they taste great, compliment all your other vegetables and they are bursting with nutrients.

They contain plenty of vitamins, including vitamin A, vitamin C, vitamin K, and Vitamin B8, and numerous minerals such as potassium, copper, iron, and manganese. As such, carrots can prevent heart disease, lower your blood pressure, and give your immune system a timely boost.

The beta-carotene in carrots, which is responsible for their orange color, is an antioxidant that helps maintain healthy skin and plays a key role in eye health.

Celery

Ah, celery, the slimmest, tallest, and leanest vegetable on the planet. Celery is certainly a great juicing vegetable that's 95% water content allows you to get lots of fresh, nutrient rich juice.

Despite its slim stature, a single stick of celery contains high amounts of vitamin K, vitamin A, vitamin C, folate, and potassium. Make sure to juice the green leaves as they have the most potassium content.

Celery juice blends well with all other vegetables and many fruits and is very refreshing over ice.

Cherries

Cherries have antibacterial, antioxidant, anti-cancer, and anti-inflammatory properties. The Ellagic Acid in cherries helps protect against cancer and the high iron count supports healthy blood. They are also high in vitamins A and C, biotin and potassium.

Cherries are high in sugar so consider this when choosing them for your juice.

Cucumber

The humble cucumber is one of the hard vegetables that you shouldn't be scared of putting into your juicer. Its high 95% water content makes it a great base juice that offers you excellent hydration benefits.

However, cucumbers also have many health benefits, including potassium, which reduces your risk of stroke, and an anti-inflammatory flavonol that plays a role in brain health along with polyphenols called lignans that may reduce risks for cancer.

They also have plenty of antioxidants such as vitamin C and beta-carotene that fight free radicals.

Cucumbers also promote skin health to make aging easier on the eyes.

Grapefruits

Grapefruits are loaded with immunity boosting vitamin C and limonene that may help women protect against breast cancer.

The soluble fiber they contain helps lower cholesterol and they add a fresh zing of fruity flavor to your vegetable juice without too much sugar.

Pink grapefruits are especially tasty.

Kale

Kale is a powerhouse of nutrition that contains the highest vegetable source of vitamin K, which supports bone health along with calcium, minerals, copper, potassium, iron, manganese, and tons of vitamins.

Kale is another member of the cruciferous family, alongside broccoli, and both are noted by the National Cancer Institute as playing a potentially key role in cancer prevention studies.

Low in calories, kale juices great and blends well with many fruits and vegetables. Kale is usually the star of the famous "green juice" that has taken the health world by storm.

Kohlrabi

Kohlrabi is a member of the Brassica family that also features cabbage, collard greens, and Brussels sprouts.

It has a mild sweet flavor and is very low in calories. It gives you lots of vitamin C for healthy immunity, and protects from chronic disease and cancer as it scavenges harmful free radicals that can roam inside the human body.

According to the National Cancer Institute, the phytochemicals in Kohlrabi, including isothiocyanates and sulforaphane may protect from prostate and colon cancers.

It is also rich in B vitamins such as niacin that helps protect the heart, along with the minerals, which include potassium, manganese, copper, calcium, iron, and phosphorus.

The green tops, like turnip greens hold key nutrients so should be juiced for the B vitamins, carotenes, vitamin-A, vitamin K, and minerals.

Juice kohlrabi with kale, carrots, apples, ginger, and lemon, which are all great complementary flavors to its lightly sweet, refreshing taste.

Lemons and Limes

You really can't go wrong with lemons. They add a citrus zing to your juice like no other fruit, as they can contribute a fresh, crisp fruity flavor to many different juice recipes.

They're also a miracle cure, as lemons have been known to help with internal bleeding, sore throats, indigestion, dental issues, respiratory disorders, high blood pressure and more.

Lemon juice in particular is super healthy, and can lower your risk of stroke, lower your body temperature if you're feeling feverish and the high vitamin C content in lemons protects your immunity and keeps that cold away.

Because many of us simply can't find ways to add lemons to our diet, juicing is the way to go. Lemons have a low sugar content and are ideal for those concerned with high sugar fruit and diabetes. Limes are also great for flavor.

Papaya

If you ever get bored of juicing pineapples, you could try papaya. They offer all the lush taste of the tropics that pineapples do, but they have much less sugar and a unique flavor.

They're nutritional powerhouses with B vitamins, vitamin C, Panthothenic acid, folate, plenty of flavonoids and much more.

Papaya's lower cholesterol, help with weight loss, boost immunity, and they are also great for your eyes. Try them!

Pineapples

Pineapples add fantastic tropical flavor to you juice blends and can help mask the flavor of vegetables for those who just can't stand the taste. This can be especially useful when you are trying to get kids to get their vegetables nutrients. They look amazing and they taste even better.

While pineapples are high in sugar, they are very beneficial to your health. They contain numerous anti-inflammatory, antibacterial, and antiviral properties, which ensure that they can cure skin ailments, prevent hair loss, strengthen your gums and bones, and they can even reduce your risk of developing certain cancers. Keep in mind that pineapples are high in sugar and should be used in moderation.

Spinach

We all saw Popeye's muscles bulge when he ate his spinach, and yet many of us never touch the stuff. If you hate eating spinach, try juicing it instead.

It is an excellent source of vitamins A, C, and E, along with calcium, iron, potassium, protein, and choline that supports healthy brain function.

It blends great with ginger, apples and carrots, and many other gems in the produce aisle.

Sweet Potatoes

For your juice to be the coolest in town, it needs a pinch of sweetness. The best way to get said sweetness is via the smoothest vegetable of them all, the suave sweet potato.

The sweet potato looks the part and tastes the part (and is indeed one of the tastiest vegetables known to man), but it also comes with lots of nutritional value, too.

It's rich in vitamin A, vitamin B6 and vitamin C, contains lots of iron and magnesium, and because their natural sugars are released slowly into your blood stream, you don't get any of those nasty spikes in your blood sugar levels.

Swiss Chard

Swiss chard is another nutritional powerhouse that is high in vitamin K, which assists with blood clotting, and protects your bones.

Moreover, you get vitamins A and C, magnesium, potassium, and iron.

If you hate eating greens, juice your chard to get all the health benefits, and it blends great with lemons, ginger, apples, or pears.

Tomatoes

Many people still get confused as to whether the tomato is a fruit or a vegetable. Tomatoes are fruits and they taste fabulous. Juicing is a great way to get more of these delicious red lovelies into your diet.

Tomatoes come with lots of health benefits; they can reduce your risk of cancer with lycopene and they promote heart health, as they are rich in vitamin C, vitamin B-6, vitamin A, and antioxidants.

They also blend well with your other fruit and vegetables, which ensure a great tasting juice. Fresh tomato juice is refreshing, and can satisfy your sweet tooth in a healthy way when you choose sweet tomatoes like Romano, grape tomatoes or the orange varieties.

Wheatgrass

Wheatgrass is one of nature's best plant foods. There is a lot of talk that wheatgrass can cure disease, prevent disease and is often over-hyped by the unregulated supplement industry as a miracle cure. Experts, like Mayo Clinic and WebMd advise that there is no scientific evidence to that effect. However, wheatgrass does provide a highly concentrated amount of a wide range of important nutrients that boost your health.

Wheatgrass is the young grass of the wheat plant that contains high amounts of chlorophyll, amino acids, calcium, enzymes, vitamins A, C, E, K, B6, riboflavin, thiamin, 92 minerals, iron, zinc, copper, manganese, and selenium.

4 grams of wheatgrass also contains 252mg or 1260% of the daily-recommended value of Niacin. Niacin or vitamin B3 is important for general good health. It is used

in medicine as a treatment to improve high cholesterol levels and reduce risks for cardiovascular disease.

According to WebMD, good evidence exists that niacin helps reduce atherosclerosis, or hardening of the heart arteries.

Wheatgrass must be drank within 15 minutes of juicing to get all its nutritional benefits. It's best undiluted and drank on an empty stomach, (as is true for most fresh juice) in order for the body to absorb all its nutrients.

Herbs and Spices

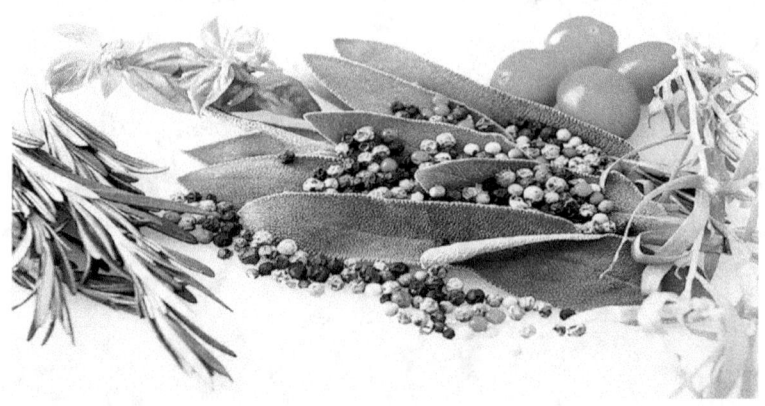

There are virtually limitless options in ways to mix up your practice of juicing, which begs the question "what herbs and spices are best?"

The base of healthy juices includes lots of vegetables, and fruits in moderation to yield a highly nutrient dense juice, but the well-timed addition of herbs and spices can push their utility over the edge, resulting in a true super drink.

However, before you just go through your pantry and select random herbs or spices without merit, you must consider their efficacy; do they actually have health benefits, or are they just tasty?

Black Pepper

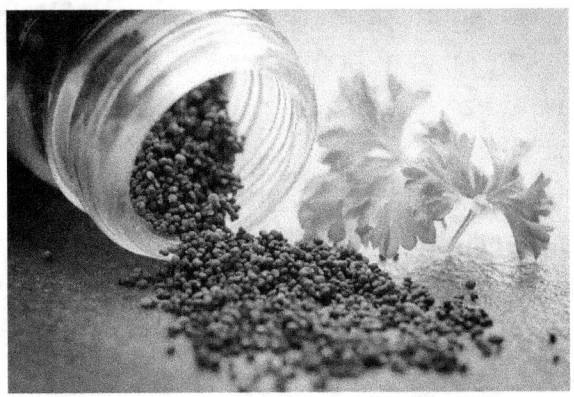

The utility of black pepper is unimaginable! Before you shrug it off and think it's too spicy for your liking, it's important to realize that you're not adding a cup of it; merely a pinch. Available virtually everywhere in the world, by incorporating a little into your daily juicing ritual, you can expect to see some of the following benefits:

- **Boosts Digestion** - when ingested, black pepper is able to stimulate the release of gastric hydrochloric acid, facilitating the breakdown of proteins and other foods. In cases of insufficient hydrochloric acid secretion, food takes a very long time to be digested, and may even transit into the intestines not well digested, resulting in bloating and possibly diarrhea.
- **Anti-Gas Agent** - though not fully understood, it is believed to be due in part to stimulating the release of hydrochloric acid (hence, lower likelihood of undigested material being target for bacterial consumption).

- **Anti-Oxidant Agent** - useful for a multitude of reasons, but primarily to combat oxidative stresses acting on our body daily. Antioxidants reduce or minimize damage caused by these oxidative particles.
- **Anti-Bacterial** - used for centuries to treat mild bacterial infections, especially when combined with other natural anti-biotics, such as honey, which, coincidentally, is added to smoothies and juices sometimes as a natural sweetener.
- **Promotes Weight Loss**- black pepper is able to increase thermogenesis, as well as stimulate the burning of fat as an energy source. It is also a mild diuretic, helping you shed excess water weight.

How to Use?

A small pinch added directly to your finished juice is all you need. It will inevitably add a slightly spicy "kick," but hardly unpleasant.

Cinnamon

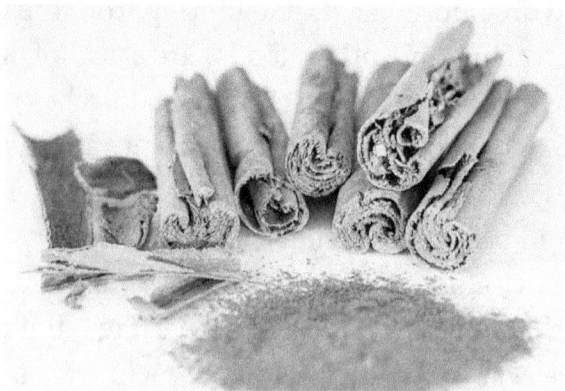

No list of super health promoting herbs or spices would be complete without the inclusion of cinnamon. Used for centuries, and maybe even millennia, its rich in calcium, magnesium, zinc and fiber, and gives food a pleasant "sweetish" taste, without being sweet itself. Cinnamon has the following well-established effects on health:

- **Anti-Oxidant Effect**- cinnamon is effective in scavenging for damaging free radical, and neutralizes them before they can harm good cells.
- **Keeps Blood Sugar Levels Stable** - cinnamon has become an important part of a diabetic's health regime, since it has consistently helped them control their blood glucose levels, and lead trouble free lives. In fact, it helps control blood sugar levels in two ways, one by improving insulin sensitivity, and two by decreasing the urge to binge on sweets. This can be very advantageous when trying to lose weight without the crash.

How to Use?

The versatility of Cinnamon enables it to be added to many different juices, and it adds a unique woody taste. It may be difficult to consume 2 grams once, so if you have juices multiple times daily, split the amount added.

Turmeric

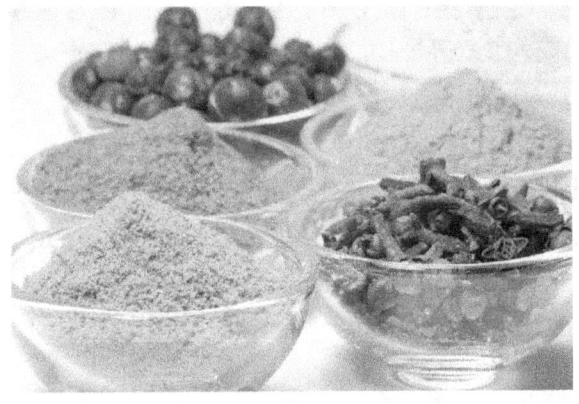

Turmeric is a versatile wonder spice that has been in use for hundreds of years in Asian cooking and by herbal medicine. This brightly colored spice is related to ginger, and is used frequently in curries and similar foods requiring lots of spice. The major health benefits of turmeric are related to its potent antioxidant ability, which has even been investigated and confirmed in scientific studies.

In fact, there is promising research that shows turmeric may play a key role in preventing cancer, as it shows immense promise in suppressing development of certain types of cancer, as well as providing support to established drugs used to treat various cancer conditions.

Consider adding it to your juices for these massive benefits:
- **Increases Levels of Brain-Derived Neurotrophic Factor** - think of this as a sort of growth hormone that functions in the brain, allowing neurons to multiply, and forms new connections, helps you preserve memory and function better cognitively. Persons with Alzheimer's or even depression have been noted to have low levels of BDNF, thus turmeric is a very likely aid.
- **Reduces Risk of Heart Disease** - turmeric helps to improve the elasticity of the blood vessel internal wall, as well as reducing levels of artery clogging plaque, decreasing the likelihood of heart attacks, strokes, or even ischemia.

- **Reduces Symptoms of Joint Pain and Arthritis** - thanks to its potent anti-inflammatory effect, suffers from joint pain may notice measurable relief in symptoms.
- **Cancer Prevention** - Numerous studies have shown curcumin, a compound found in turmeric to have substantial benefits in reducing risk for cancer.

How to Use?

Fresh turmeric can be juiced along with your other fruits and vegetables. Alternatively, you can add 1 or 2 teaspoons of the dry spice to 1 glass of juice daily to. It will dye your beverage slightly yellow but a small price to pay for bountiful health...right?

Ginger

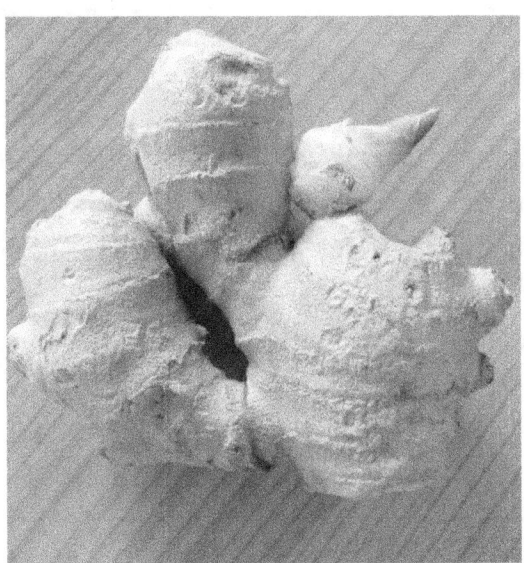

If you grew up with your grandma, you undoubtedly know the merits of adding ginger to your food... but maybe not the convenience of adding it to juice or smoothies! In fact, if you suffer from any intestinal issues, or heartburn, ginger will quickly become a go to in your arsenal, and no- it's not acidic, as people believe.

This wonder-spice can help you out in a pinch with the following:

- **Reduces Nausea or Vomiting** - if you suffer from chronic acid reflux, quite often nausea accompanies it. Consuming a little ginger, either juiced in fresh form or grated into a powder and added to your finished juice blend will help.
- **May Improve Blood Sugar and Decrease Risk of Heart Disease** - this is a relatively new area of study, but appears very promising. Over the course of a 12-week study, daily consumption of 2 grams of ginger daily delivered massive improvements in blood sugar levels, along with markers for cardiac health. The more markers you are positive for, the higher your likelihood of having a serious cardiac event in the coming years.
- **Helps Treat Gingival Disease** - how about swishing around your juice in your mouth before drinking? As weird as it sounds, that's exactly another way to juice the benefits of ginger (pun intended). Ginger inhibits the growth of bacteria implicated in the development of oral disease, so maybe can be utilized instead of Listerine, who knows?

How Much Ginger Should Be Added to Juices?

If you're going to be juicing the ginger root itself, a 1-inch sized piece is sufficient. However, if you will be grating and adding it directly to juices, half of a teaspoon is sufficient. Ginger may seem extremely spicy to some, so if required start with less and gradually build appreciation for the taste.

Cilantro

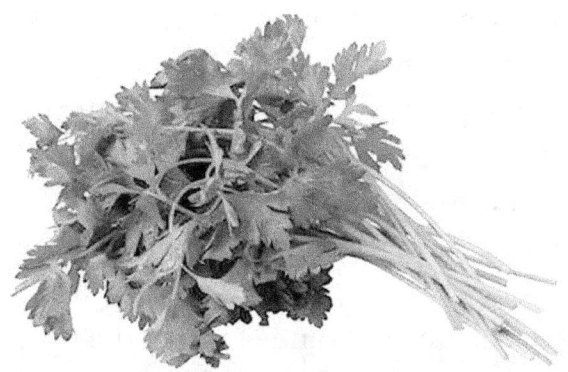

Cilantro is a powerful vegetable to add to your juice. It is great at detoxing. And check out the following health benefits:

- Powerful anti-inflammatory capacities that may help symptoms of arthritis
- Protective agents against bacterial infection from Salmonella in food products
- Acts to increase HDL cholesterol (the good kind), and reduces LDL cholesterol (the bad kind)
- Relief for stomach gas, prevention of flatulence and an overall digestive aid
- Wards off urinary tract infections
- Helps reduce feelings of nausea
- Eases hormonal mood swings associated with menstruation
- Has been shown to reduce menstrual cramping.
- Adds fiber to the digestive tract

- A source of iron, magnesium, and is helpful in fighting anemia
- Gives relief for diarrhea, especially if caused by microbial or fungal infections
- Helps promote healthy liver function.
- Reduces minor swelling
- Strong general antioxidant properties
- Disinfects and helps detoxify the body
- Stimulates the endocrine glands
- Helps with insulin secretion and lowers blood sugar
- Acts as a natural anti-septic and anti-fungal agent for skin disorders like fungal infections and eczema
- Contains immune-boosting properties
- Acts as an expectorant
- Helps ease conjunctivitis, as well as eye-aging, macular degeneration, and other stressors on the eyes.

Cumin

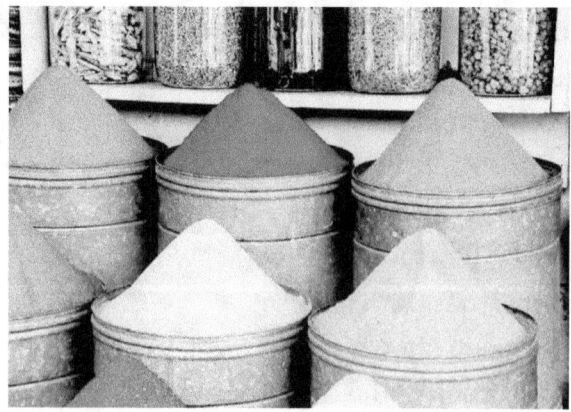

An ancient spice used for centuries in the Far East, this seed is a staple of Indian diets around the world, and is typically consumed roasted. It has numerous health benefits, and is great to add to your juices:

Benefits of consuming cumin and adding to juices include:

- **Boosts Digestion** - the oil that gives cumin its aromatic smell is known as Cuminaldehyde, and kick starts the digestive process by stimulating salivary output. Next, is a compound called thymol, which then bolsters the production of salivary secretions and enzymes, ensuring that your food is well digested and subsequently absorbed.

- **Relieves Respiratory Conditions** - surprisingly to most, cumin acts as a mild expectorant, being able to break up mucus and relieve bronchial congestion. The presence of aromatic oils also helps to expel and loosen mucus, which also possess disinfectant properties to reduce bacterial load and possible infection.

- **Helps Treat Anemia** - cumin is rich in iron, which promotes healthy development of red blood cells. It also improves symptoms of low energy, and chronic fatigue as oxygen carrying potential of blood is increased.

- **May Help Prevent Cancer** - has significant anti-cancer and detoxifying properties, via boosting secretion of enzymes that destroy abnormal cells. It is also rich in vitamins A and C, which are proven anti-oxidants useful in combating cancer promoting free radicals.

How Much Cumin Should I Use?

Taking just one teaspoon per day, most likely ground and incorporated into your juices is the easiest way. Cumin will likely add an exotic taste to your vegetable-based juices, so get ready to set your taste buds alight!

Nutmeg

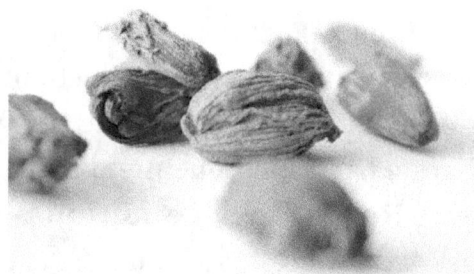

One of the most flavorful spices in the world, nutmeg is actually a seed that is still loaded with nutritional and health benefits. It is rich in fiber, B vitamins, magnesium, copper, and fiber.

By adding a bit of this powdered spice to your juices, you can reap the health benefits outlined below:

- **May Help Relieve Pain** - nutmeg functions in a way similar to menthol in how it relieves pain. It is also helpful in relieving inflammatory conditions, as well as smooth muscle pain (abdominal or organ pain).
- **Works Well in Managing Oral Health** - nutmeg is very effective in killing bacteria found in the mouth, which may be responsible for embarrassing bad breath or more serious

conditions such as gingivitis. In fact, many mouthwash products include nutmeg by virtue of its effectiveness.

- **Treats Sleeplessness** - thanks to its high magnesium content, nutmeg has been used historically to relieve nerves and induce sleep.
- **Treating Pediatric Leukemia** - interestingly, nutmeg has shown promise in treating this debilitating disease, which primarily affects children. Its essential oils and methanol like constituent has led to cancer cells committing suicide, a process known as apoptosis.
- **Improves Blood Pressure** - minerals contained in nutmeg have known vasodilatory effects, which allow blood vessels to expand and reduce the pressure in them, and subsequent strain on the heart.

How Much Nutmeg Should Be Added to Your Juice?

A teaspoon of the ground powder added to your juice is sufficient. It will improve taste significantly, as well as offer great insurance against illness. It is important not to overdose on nutmeg consumption, as there have been reports of people trying to get "high" from its euphoric rush following over dosage. And, of course, deaths followed.

Parsley

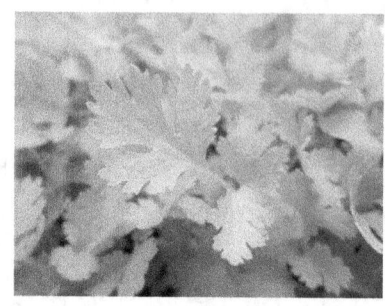

A popular herb used for its leaves since the days of Roman domination. Typically, many people now use parsley for garnishing, but it's far more useful when grated or juiced and added to other nutritional powerhouses to make a strong healthy blend.

Parsley has demonstrated several benefits on health, including the following:

- **Boosts Immune Function** - parsley is reportedly able to increase T cell count, and bolster the action of lymphocytes, thanks to its many bioactive nutrients.
- **Anti- Inflammatory and Detoxifying Properties** - parsley aids in treatment and management of many inflammatory processes, such as arthritis and interestingly even liver inflammation and jaundice. By helping return elevated liver enzymes to normal, detoxification of toxins resumes and health improves.
- **Eases diarrhea**
- **Helps to eliminate excess water from your system (weight loss)**

Mint

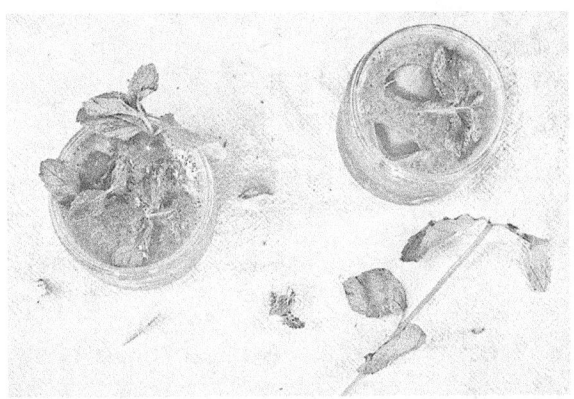

Mint gives a fresh kick to anything it's added to, and also delivers health benefits to boot. If you've never experienced the health benefits of mint, you might be surprised as how many there are:

- **Boosts Digestion** - mint leaves have an established track record of soothing indigestion and helping relieve acid heartburn. Is it any coincidence that many antacids come in mint flavor?

- **May Help Reduce Asthma Symptoms** - mint is a useful bronchodilator, relieves chest congestion, and can soothe the airways. However, too much can likely be an irritant to the same organs.

- **Boosts The Immune System** - especially useful in persons with seasonal allergies, regular consumption of mint helps to modulate the release of histamine, which signals the start of allergic reactions.

- **May Decrease Likelihood of Cancer** - different from making use of anti-oxidants, enzymes contained in mint may help prevent the development of cancer, at least when consumed as part of a healthy lifestyle.

- **Headaches and Nausea** - mint has been classically used to relieve headaches and upset feelings, and is still used and recommended across the world as a safe, non-drowsy alternative to other products.

How Should Mint Be Added to Juices?

You can either add a few mint leaves to your juicer, or add drops of 100% pure mint extract to finished juices. Either way, you will have a refreshing, energizing juice loaded with beneficial health boosters!

Basil

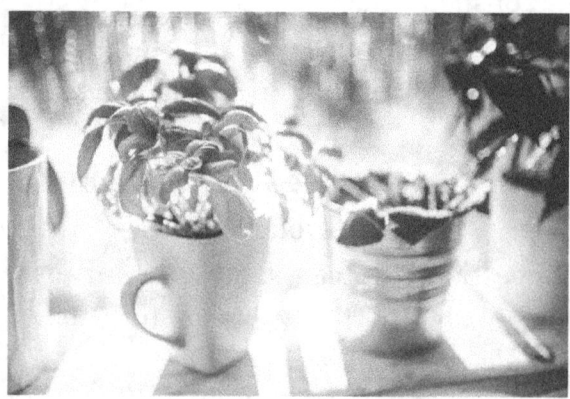

Basil or Ocimum basilicum, also referred to as Saint Joseph's Wort, is an herb that belongs to the mint family Lamiaceae. This aromatic and pungent herb is native to India and other tropical areas of Asia.

The International journal of Agronomy and Plant Production, states that the word Basil is derived from the Greek word "basileus" that means "king" and the Oxford

English Dictionary states that this herb was likely used as some type of medicine or royal unguent.

Basil is often used in traditional Tamil and Ayurvedic medicine, and Jewish folklore believes basil to give strength during fasting.

The most commercially available type of basil and one used widely in Italian cooking is Sweet basil, and it has a very strong clove scent and flavor. Lime and lemon basil has a strong citrus flavor that comes from its high concentration of limonene.

Health Benefits of Basil

- **Powerful Antioxidants** - One study conducted at Purdue University (Juliani, H.R. and J.E. Simon et al) found basil to contain a wide range of health boosting essential oils that are rich in phenolic compounds and polyphenol antioxidants, flavonoids and anthocyanins. Basil extract was shown to have more antioxidant activity than standard antioxidants found in vegetables and fruits, a fact documented in a study that was published in the Journal of Advanced Pharmacy Education & Research.

- **Anti-inflammatory** - This flavorful herb contains compounds that might be helpful in treating inflammatory bowel diseases and arthritis (J Gertsch et al).

- **Anti-aging** - Research presented at the British Pharmaceutical Conference demonstrated that basil could improve the aging process and reduce its harmful effects. Holy basil extract was successfully used to kill of harmful molecules and curtail the typical damage that occurs from free radicals in the heart, brain and other vital organs.

- **Nutrient Rich** - Bails is also nutrient rich and contains vitamin A, K, and C, iron, calcium, magnesium, and potassium.

Basil is very easy to grow in small containers placed on a sunny window sill, so you can enjoy the fresh herb whenever you juice.

How to Juice Basil

Thoroughly wash the leaves and remove grit from between the leaves. Tear off the leaves, roll them up into a tight bunch, and push through your juice with firmer produce, like apples or kale.

Final Thoughts

The taste boost that they provide to sometimes horrible tasting juices is another major perk and can help ensure you remain compliant in getting your recommended dose of nutrients every day.

Think of herbs and spices quite simply as nature's tiny gifts to us, to spruce up the foods we consume, and keep our body functioning optimally.

On a final note, do not be intimidated trying to add as many herbs and spices as you can to your juices. It's perfectly fine to choose just a few at the beginning, learn what taste you appreciate best, and also consider which benefit you are most looking forward to.

Juicing Tips

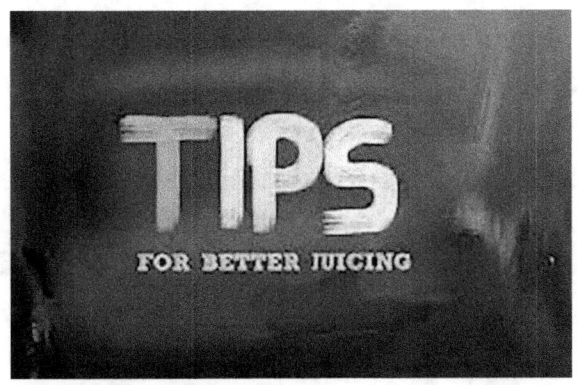

Juicing Facts and Myths

People who juice are often faced with questions from others who do not understand the benefits of juices. Here are some facts and myths about juicing that you will want to consider:

- **Juice has no fiber in it.** This is a myth. Juice contains plenty of soluble fiber that soaks up glucose and cholesterol, lowering the amounts of these substances in the bloodstream. Soluble fiber also takes on water so the stool is bulked up and bowel movements are easier.

- **Juices contain a lot of sugar.** This can be partially true because some juices contain fruit sugar. This is why many experts on juicing advise a ratio of 80% vegetables to 20% fruit, which allows you to add a bit of sweetness along with all the sugar free benefits of found in vegetables.

- **You can't detoxify on juice.** This is partially true. While vegetables like broccoli, cauliflower, kale, radishes, cabbage, and Brussels sprouts have phytonutrients in them that increase the enzymes in the liver, it is the liver that does the detoxifying. We naturally detoxify ourselves every day, but adding more phytonutrients from juicing to our diets can help.

- **You can kick start a healthy diet or weight loss plan with juicing.** This is absolutely true. Juicing is a great way to detox off junk food, get your body in touch with real nutrition, and kick start your way into a healthy lifestyle.

- **Juicing has no health benefits.** Increasing research studies have shown that drinking vegetable juices will provide you with many health benefits. For example, beet juice can help manage hypertension. There are more and more studies pointing to the health benefits of juicing.

- **Juicing doesn't have protein in it.** You can add many sources of protein to your juice as you are making them. For example, you can add hemp seeds, chia seeds, or a protein powder to the juice for an added boost of protein.

- **Juice diets are just a fad.** This is another myth as juicing has only seen steady growth since the 1980's as people take heed to the lasting health benefits of increasing plant food intake to prevent disease, boost energy and improve overall health and wellness. Carrot juice, for example, has been shown through research to decrease the damage to WBCs in smoking clients.

- **The nutrients leave the juice in the extracted pulp.** This is another myth. When you juice, only the insoluble fiber is removed with the pulp, but many vital micronutrients remain in the juice along with soluble fiber making it a very healthy beverage.

- **It is better to eat fruits and vegetables than it is to juice them.** This is partly true if you are looking for a source of insoluble fiber. The other nutrients in juice can be found whether 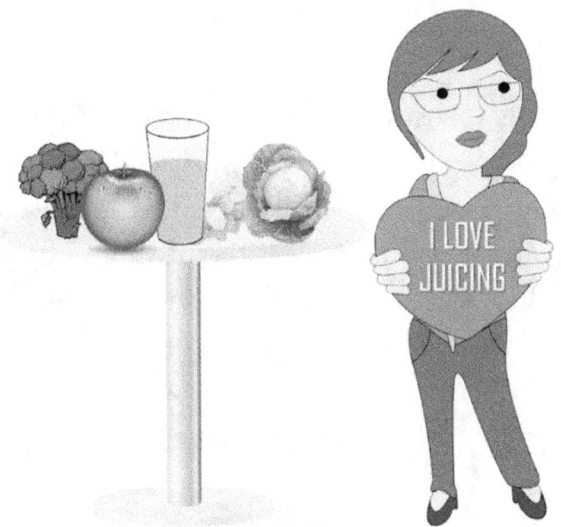 you eat the vegetable (or fruit) or drink them in juice form. Some vegetables are actually healthier for you in a juice when compared to roasting or otherwise cooking them.

- **Juices can be contaminated with bacteria.** You can get bacteria in juice but it is usually in the manufactured form of juices and not in the juice, you make at home. Wash your hands before you make your juice, peel vegetables before juicing, and wash the vegetables before putting them in the juicer. Drink them right away or store them in the refrigerator for no longer than 72 hours.

- **You can lose your hair if you juice.** This is only true if you have an underlying medical condition, such as hypothyroidism. If you are worried that you might have a condition that leads to hair loss, talk to your doctor before starting a juicing program. Make sure the juice has health-retaining nutrients in it, such as zinc, protein, and biotin.
- **Juicing is much too expensive.** While you do have to invest in a juicer, you should know that it is not much more expensive to juice your vegetables and fruits than it is to eat them whole. If you don't want to waste anything, you can save the pulp for use in soups, cookies, and in other baked goods.

Juicing Tips for Beginners

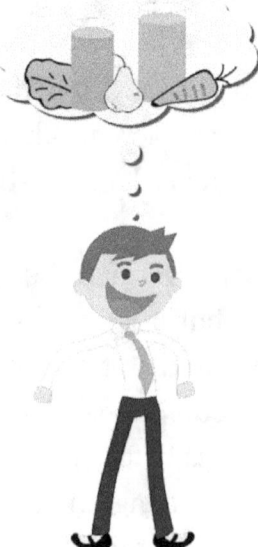

It helps to know a few things before you get started on the juicing journey, as knowledge is power.

Experiment - First of all, you can juice pretty much any type of fruit or vegetables. Don't be scared to experiment. Just think "the more the merrier." As you walk through the supermarket, consider trying something you never have before.

Get a grocery list started - Get out your recipes and make a list of all the ingredients you will need. Planning makes it much easier to juice when you need to.

Prepare your vegetables and fruits the night before a morning juicing session. This means washing the produce, peeling them if needed, and storing them overnight in airtight containers.

Nuts and Seeds - You should never juice nuts, grains or seeds, but instead grind them and add stir them into your ready-made juice. Adding nuts and seeds is a great way to boost the nutritional value of the juice and get many health benefits, but remember a little goes a long way.

Protein Powders - Protein powder can be added to juices when you drink them as a meal replacement so you get the protein you need.

Choose organic – Organic produce is more expensive, unless you buy from local farms when available, but you will ingest less pesticide and more nutrients.

Timing is everything when it comes to juicing. You don't want to be drinking your healthy fresh juice on a full stomach! If you do, your body just won't absorb all those lovely nutrients as well and some of them may even go to waste. A juice is best drank on an empty stomach. It's not going to fill you completely, but it will give your body a great chance to absorb all that goodness. Then, you can sit down to a meal an hour later.

Don't drink too quickly - this puts a LOT of pressure on your digestive enzymes that have to work extra hard to digest juice that is frank too fast. The best way to drink juice is to sit back and relax. Take care of your stomach and digestive tract because they are really sensitive.

Thoroughly wash your produce - This removes bacteria and some of the pesticide residue if you did not buy organic. This is especially important with leafy greens where dirt can be stuck in between the leaves.

Line the pulp basket in the juicer - If your juicer has a pulp basket, you will need to line it with a plastic bag. This makes cleaning up the juicer afterward much easier.

Cut the produce so it fits - You can tear up the greens or cut up the larger vegetables so that it fits through the feeding chute of the juicer.

Read your juicer's user manual – This is very important because you will learn best practices for cutting produce, and also which speeds should be used for which fruits and vegetables. This will not only yield you the best juice, but will prevent breakage of the machine. For example, usually harder vegetables are best juiced on high, while softer vegetables, such as cabbage and spinach, are best juiced on a lower setting.

Rerun the pulp - In order to get the most nutrients out of the juice, take out the pulp, and run it through the juicer again to get more juice from the damp, left over pulp.

Clean the juicer right after use - You should do this right away so as to keep bacteria from building up inside the juicer. If it is dishwasher safe, you can put those parts in the dishwasher. Otherwise, you should scrub the juicer out with hot or warm water and a mild dish soap.

Allow the juicer to dry on a drying mat rather than drying it out with a towel as this can get towel fibers in your next batch of juice.

Drink your juice while its fresh - The nutrients will go away if you keep the juice sitting too long and also remember that this is not store bought juice full of preservatives so it will not keep fresh as long. Put any leftover juice in a glass or BPA-free plastic airtight container in the refrigerator for no longer than 3 days.

Tips for Storing Juice

- If you are making a double batch, separate the batches and put the juice you are not drinking in the refrigerator right way.
- Fill the container to the top. You want to have as little space in the container as possible. If you have too much space, the oxygen in the container will begin to destroy the delicate micronutrients.
- If you want to freeze your juice, make sure you do so immediately after juicing, and for no longer than 7 to 10 days.

Avoiding The Sugar Trap

Fruit contain much more sugar than vegetables and some fruits contain much more than others do. Some fruits are very high in sugar, a count that gets even higher when the fruit is juiced, so that fact can negate any benefits they might have. In fact, sugar content is key when considering fruits in your new juicing lifestyle.

Some have so much sugar that you might want to use them in moderation or avoid them altogether, especially if you don't want a spike in your blood sugar levels if you have diabetes or weight issues, and definitely if you are juicing for weight loss.

Experts always tell us to eat more fruit and vegetables. What they don't really go into detail on is the fact that some fruits can actually be harmful when consumed in excess.

This is where juicing can become a problem.

Consider the fact that in order to get about 2 ounces of orange juice, you need to juice 2 medium oranges, so for a regular 6-ounce glass of juice, that is 3 oranges.

One medium orange has 12 grams of sugar and 62 calories, so when you drink that 6-ounce juice you just ingested 36 grams of sugar and 186 calories just from one drink!

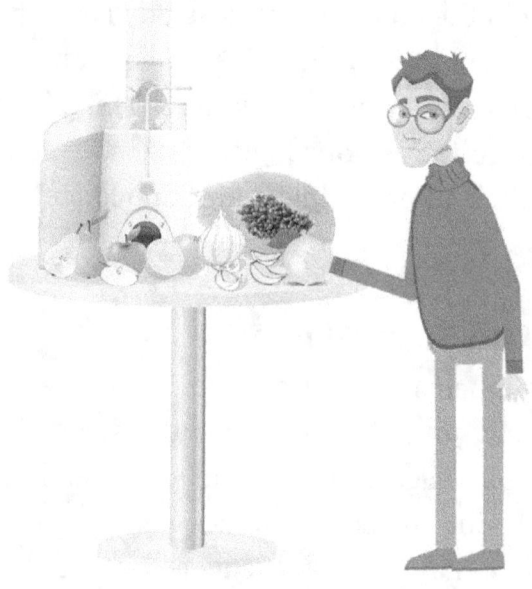

Now, consider if you have or ever will eat 3 oranges in one sitting? You likely would not, so the point is that when you are juicing fruit, you can easily send your sugar and calorie intake through the roof.

Moreover, this is one of the pitfalls to watch out for when starting your juicing journey. People love the sweet taste of fruit juice, and because it's juicing they automatically assume that it's all healthy, but when you look at the sugar and calorie intake, you can see how quickly this healthy habit can turn ugly for those who drink that 6-ounce orange juice, 2, 3 or 4 times a day!

By the way, US federal dietary guidelines recommend that adults eat 1 1/2 to 2 cups of fruit daily, which is about 2 oranges.

While the sugar from fruit is better for you than table sugar because you are also getting the nutrients that fruit has to offer and not just empty calories as the cupcake does, in excess it can it can harm you just as that cupcake can by contributing to weight gain and increasing risks for type 2 diabetes.

If You Only Juice Fruits, You're Really Missing the Point of Juicing

If You Mostly Juice Fruits, You Are Missing the Point of Juicing

The fruit should always be used in moderation to complement and enhance the flavor of vegetables that are the star ingredients in all your juice blends.

50 Tips to Juice Like a Pro

1. Make a commitment to juicing and stick to it, this can be tricky if you are not used to the practice but with time, dedication and regular use it can become so deeply embedded that it will simply be something you won't want to live without. It can take several weeks to form a solid juicing habit, so stick with it and make sure to juice regularly.

2. Create a juicing schedule. Make plans depending on how much your juicer can juice at one time, how much prep is necessary for produce, and how much

time you can dedicate each day or every other day to be sure that you have fresh juice available at all times.

3. Stick with a regular juicing schedule to support the habit. Studies show that consumption of large doses of specific vitamins, minerals, and enzymes can aid in the prevention and management of symptoms associated with heart disease, cancer, and strokes and can strengthen immunity against colds and flu, increase bone density and improve the condition of the skin. We know that studies have shown that it is recommended that we consume six to eight servings of vegetables and fruits daily. This can be challenging for many people, juicing ensures that you reach the recommended daily intake for vegetables in a convenient manner.

4. Buy a quality juicer - many vegetables, like beets and carrots, are actually quite difficult to pulverize
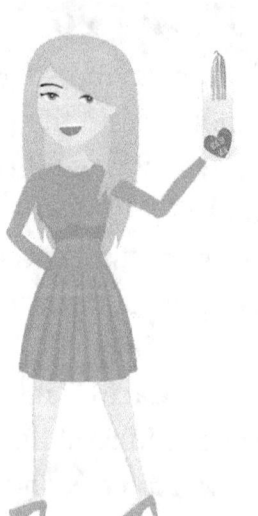
properly, and cheap juicers will not do the job. Buying a juicer that is powerful enough to pulverize efficiently and rapidly is one of the keys to buying a great juicer. If you plan to juice a lot of hard vegetables, your best choice is a centrifugal juicer.

5. If you plan to juice mostly greens, then consider a masticating juicer that is great for greens and also supplies a high juice yield.

6. Consider the size of the mixing container. If you go too small, you'll only be able to juice a little at a time, so make sure you invest in a unit that has the capacity for your juicing needs. This is especially important for large families.

7. Keep a produce shopping list to stay organized and have all the ingredients you need at hand when you want to juice.

8. If you plan to juice in the morning, then prep your produce as needed the night before. This is especially useful when your mornings are rushed or time limited.

9. Always wash produce thoroughly to eliminate all dirt particles, and some of the pesticides when not buying organic produce. This is especially important with leafy greens where dirt hides between the leaves.

10. Line your juicer's pulp basket with a plastic bag for easy clean up.

11. Juice every day to build a healthy habit. When daily juicing is not possible, you can store juice in the fridge in an airtight container for up to 3 days.

12. Juice vegetables that you do not normally eat. Every vegetable provides a different benefit to the

body but everyone is different in terms of what vegetables they enjoy eating, and so they skip those they don't like due to either taste, smell or texture. Juicing these allows you to obtain benefits from vegetables that you would not ordinarily consume, and since you can mask their taste with fruit, lemons, ginger and other enhancers getting these nutrients becomes much less of a burden.

13. Consider sugar content of fruits when you juice, as some have so much sugar they should be consumed 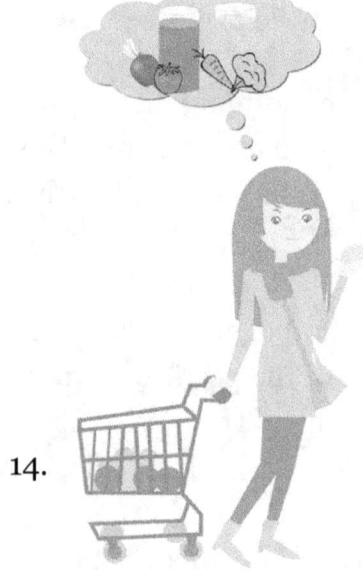 in moderation or avoided altogether, especially for those who need to avoid spikes in blood sugar levels (diabetics), those with weight issues, and definitely those who are juicing for weight loss.

14. Taste as you go and adjust accordingly, just as you would during cooking.

15. Consuming juices first thing in the morning or at any time when your stomach is empty will optimize the rate at which the vitamins, minerals, antioxidants, and enzymes are absorbed and used by the body. It also gives you a great energy boost to kick-start your day with the drive you need.

Additionally, consuming raw fruit and vegetables provides an intensive boost of vitamins and enzymes, which are directed straight to the blood stream. This means that your digestive system does not need to process the fruit and vegetables as they would if you were to consume them whole.

16. Juice high water vegetables, like cucumbers and broccoli. People often struggle with reaching the recommended daily intake of water. With six to eight glasses being the goal, some find it difficult to reach this intake. Many juicing combinations incorporate an element of water as the basis for the recipe, and indeed many vegetables and fruits have a high water concentration, meaning that you are extracting water during the juicing process. Juicing provides a great strategy for increasing your water intake each day to hydrate your body.

17. Make sure to juice vegetables with fruit. If you only consume fruit based juices, your intake of sugar and calories will be unnecessarily high. By integrating vegetable juicing into your daily diet, you will be able to optimize the volume of vitamins, minerals, antioxidants, and enzymes being absorbed by your body.

18. Make sure that you follow the 80/20 rule when it comes to the ratio of vegetables to fruit. 80% vegetables that will give you the immunity, wellness, and energy boost you need and 20% fruit

for more nutrients and taste. So, add an apple to give some sweetness or an orange if you crave some zesty citrus flavor.

19. Make sure that you include one or two root vegetables in your juicing combination. By adding in a carrot or beet into your recipe, you will be able to give the juice an intense boost of antioxidants, while also gaining a sweet but earthy flavor, which makes it more palatable when drinking.

20. To optimize the nutritional properties of your juice you need to ensure that you include a minimum of at least, one leafy green vegetable such as kale, broccoli, or chard, which will give you an enormous amount of unique nutrients.

21. 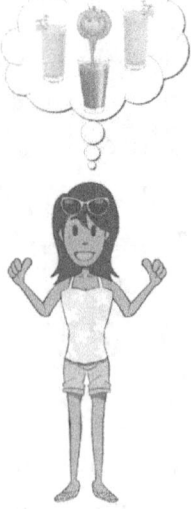 High water content vegetables such as a cucumbers or celery will assist in diffusing the very (and sometimes overpowering) flavors of kale, broccoli, or chard, which help to ensure that the juice you prepare is easy to drink.

22. Add some kind of garnish to not only provide a concentrated

54

and intensive vitamin boost but also to make the juice really tasty. Great options include, ginger, lemons, limes or mint.

23. Re-juice any still wet pulp to get the most bang for your juicing buck.

24. Juice to improve the aging process - as we age our ability to digest what we need can become impaired as our organs work less optimally. By preparing food in this liquid and raw form, it becomes "pre-digested" which means that the body can absorb the vitamins, minerals, antioxidants and enzymes quickly and most efficiently.

25. Juicing fruit alone greatly increases your sugar intake, which can lead to weight gain and erratic blood sugar spikes that actually stimulate hunger, negating the positive benefits that juicing offers.

26. Include lots of vegetables in your juicing to benefit from chlorophyll, which is a compound that acts as the life force within the plant. This compound also offers significant beneficial properties for humans. Consumed raw as part of a juicing regime, the chlorophyll is digested straight into your bloodstream meaning that you are getting all of the benefits that the vegetables have to offer. Wheatgrass has the highest amount of chlorophyll.

27. Drink more green juice. Green juice is juice made mostly from dark leafy greens, such as kale, broccoli, and spinach, but can also include celery, cabbage, broccoli, and apples. Green juice is your best choice in a highly nutrient rich and low sugar drink.

28. For some, the perception that green colored juice looks bad and therefore tastes bad can interfere with the healthy practice of juicing. You can get past your perceived dislike for the color of the juice by adding in some red berries or orange carrots that will improve the color and taste to get a boost of vitamins, minerals, antioxidants and enzymes that you need to optimize your mental and physical health and wellbeing.

29. To help you become acclimated to the taste of vegetable juice, ease yourself into the taste of green vegetable 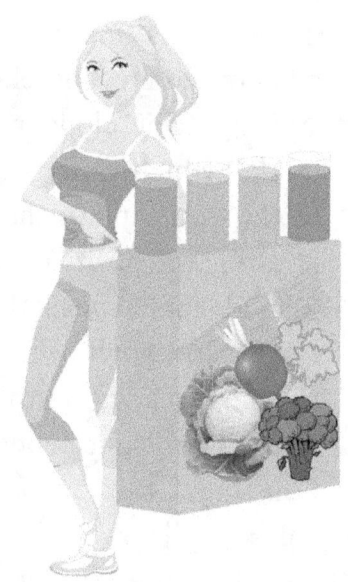 -based juices so that you aren't immediately repelled and become turned off juicing forever. Start with mild-tasting vegetables such as celery and cucumbers. As you start to build your juicing palette, you can start to incorporate lettuce, kale, spinach, parsley, or cilantro.

30. To counteract that bitterness of vegetable and green juices, you can add in elements of lemon or

lime, grapefruits, cranberries or ginger, each of which have excellent properties that are associated with health and wellbeing.

31. Continue to eat whole vegetables and fruits even while juicing as they produce important insoluble fiber that your body needs.

32. It is best to consume juice on an empty stomach. This will give your body an optimum energy boost and allow for optimal digestion of all of the vitamins, minerals, antioxidants and enzymes that you need to go about your day.

33.   Engage the whole family in juicing, as this is a great way to increase vegetable intake in young kids who hate eating them to make sure they benefit from the regular consumption of vitamins, minerals, antioxidants, and enzymes.

34. Collect juicing recipes, but also create your own blends to find combinations that please your palate and allow you to remain positive about your new habit.

35. To improve the health and vitality of your skin try combining cucumbers and a small apple (for taste).

36. To fight aging, choose a juicing combination that includes water/milk/aloe-vera juice, blueberries, strawberries, kale, and beetroot.

37. To enhance your libido, you can combine coconut water, celery, banana, ginger, basil, and figs.

38. To give yourself an energy boost juice a combination that includes cucumbers, celery, kale, spinach, parsley, lemon and ginger.
39. To satisfy your sweet tooth juice a combination that includes apples, celery, and stir in a little cinnamon.
40. To boost your immune system and prevent the cold and flu, juice blends that include beetroot, carrots, celery, broccoli, garlic, ginger, lemon, and cayenne   pepper.

41. If you are overworked or feeling the effects of stress in your life, prepare a stress relief juice with spinach, broccoli, celery, and carrots.
42. If you want to improve your gut health and digestion, boost your intake of papain, which is an enzyme found in papaya that helps digest proteins. Try a juice that includes papaya, kale, cabbage, ginger, and lemon.
43. Juice organic produce - Use only organic vegetables to avoid toxins, and to increase the nutritional value of your produce and healthy enzyme   intake.

44. Enhance your juices with ground nuts and seeds and protein powders. Adding protein powder to your juice makes for a great meal replacement juice.

45. Beware of long term juice cleanses, and make sure to ask your doctor before starting any sort of juice fast.

46. Engage your kids in the juicing process. Let them pick out their own ingredients to get them excited about fruits and vegetables.

47. Buy an airtight container so you can refrigerate your juice and also take it with you to work, the gym or while running errands.

48. If you have an adversity to the taste of vegetable juice, don't worry, for many it is an acquired taste. Once your body starts to feel the health benefits you'll be hooked.

49. Balance high yield produce like celery, tomatoes, apples, and cucumbers, with a low yield vegetable like kale to get more juice in your glass.

50. Use herbs and spices in your juice, including basil, parsley, cilantro, mint, turmeric, cumin, nutmeg, ginger and hot peppers to not only enhance flavor but to get their numerous health benefits.

Juicing for Specific Benefits

Juicing for Weight Loss

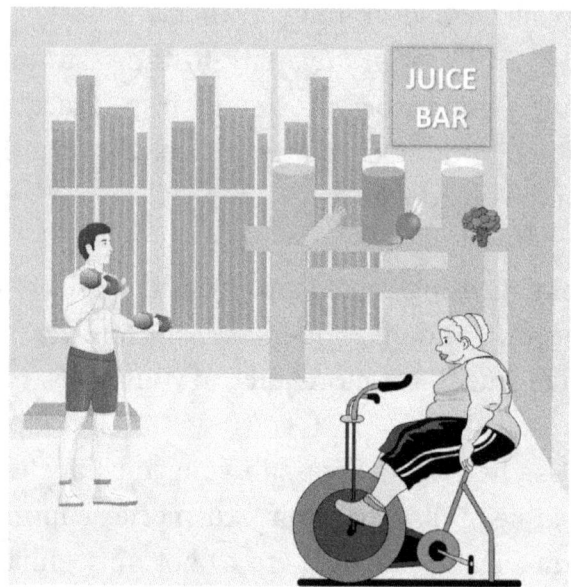

Many use juicing to lose weight, but in order to get the best results, it is important to do it right, here are ten key considerations when juicing for weight loss.

1. **Choose organic:** Use only organic vegetables to avoid toxins, and to increase the nutritional value of your produce and healthy enzyme intake.

2. **Stretch your budget:** Buy from local organic farms and in season vegetables and fruits whenever possible, as they are cheaper and certainly fresher,

allowing you to get the most from your juicing dollars.

3. **Watch your sugar intake:** Before you push that fruit through your juicer, STOP and consider this. Fruit is very high in sugar, and you can easily go into a calorie and sugar overload with just a couple of glasses a day, negating your weight loss efforts and the whole point of juicing. One example is the 1-cup of spinach that has only 7 calories and no sugar versus a large orange that has 87 calories and 17 grams of sugar. Make your juices primarily from vegetables and add sweetness and flavor with low sugar fruits like berries, lemons, limes and small amounts of green apples. Ginger is also a great way to add flavor with little calories.

4. **Stick with power vegetables:** Kale, spinach, broccoli, cabbage, greens, celery, cucumbers, and tomatoes are some of your key superfoods for juicing.

5. **Stay active and exercise:** Being active and getting regular exercise is important for weight loss as it allows you to build lean muscle mass, boost metabolism and burn more calories.

6. **Research recipes:** There are hundreds of juice recipes online and in books, and you can benefit from these tried and true blends to get the most flavor and satisfaction from your juice.

7. **Watch out for juice fast pitfalls:** According to the University of Pittsburgh Medical Center, drastic restriction of caloric intake slows metabolism that can actually make it harder to lose weight. Losing

weight too quickly on juice fasts that are too low in calories can cause you to lose more water and muscle than fat, and will likely result in regaining the weight you lost or more. Instead, use juicing to increase your intake of energy boosting nutrient rich vegetables, especially if you are a person whose diet lacks them and to detox off junk food.

8. **Add boosters to your juice:** Add ground chia or 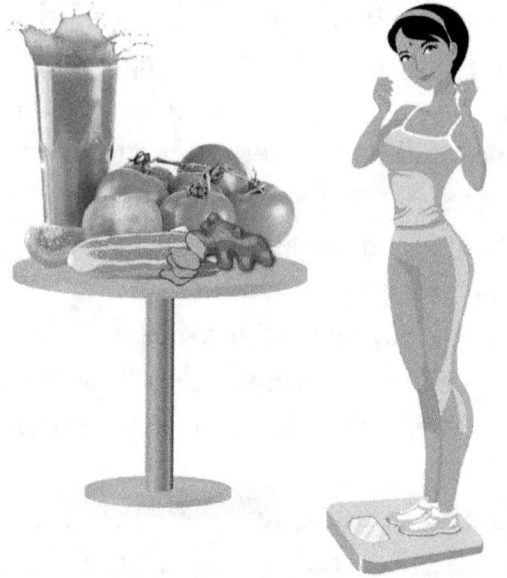 flax seeds to your juice, they are nutrient

powerhouses that fortify your juice heart-healthy omega-3 fatty acids also found in walnuts. Add protein or whey powder when using juice as a meal replacement to make you feel full longer, feed, and promote lean muscle mass and increase intake of lean protein in your diet.

9. **Eat a balanced diet:** As great as juices are for your health, they are no replacement for whole food. Many people new to juicing attempt to substitute too many meals with juice, which does

not supply enough calories to keep you fueled throughout the day, or enough fiber or other nutrients to keep you satisfied and healthy. This can lead to fatigue and hunger, which can quickly lead you to abandon your weight loss efforts. Eating a balanced diet also ensures that you meet all your nutrient needs and not go into starvation mode.

Don't fall for juicing hype: Yes, juicing is a great tool for your weight loss arsenal, but it is not a magic pill for weight loss. Learning to eat right and making profound dietary and lifestyle habit changes is key to long-term weight management success.

Juicing for Exercise

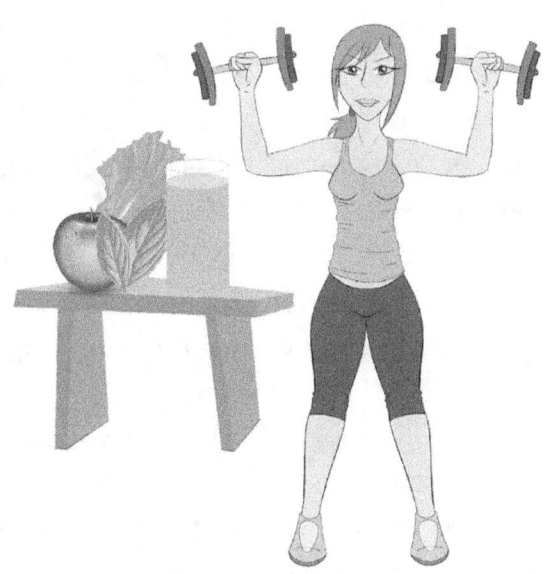

The Role of Nutrition in Exercise

Perhaps you already know that what you eat is really important. But what you're perhaps looking to learn is why when you eat is so important too - especially if you exercise.

If you drink the right nutrient-stuffed juice an hour or two before exercise and follow it up with another an hour or two after your exercise, you're pretty much meeting all your workout nutrition needs. You don't really need anything else.

However, it can also depend on what you're looking to get out of your workout. If, for example you're an endurance athlete who trains every day for high-level competition, you'll need more carbs and calories than the average person who exercises. You also need more protein.

On the other hand, maybe you're training as a bodybuilder who lifts weights in order to seriously grow muscles. Because you're looking to gain more weight, you'll need more protein and carbs. Alternatively, you may be looking to get ready for a fitness competition, in which case your cab intake should be reduced.

It also comes down to your body type. If you have an **ectomorph**, you'll probably be looking to gain more muscle. If you have a **mesomorph**, you'll probably be looking to optimize your physique. If you have an **endomorph**, you'll probably be looking to lose body fat.

However, it all comes down to the same thing: We all need nutrients to power us through a workout, and juicing them is just plain easier and faster than eating them.

Pre-Workout Nutrition

What and **when** we eat before we workout can often make a huge different to not only your performance, but also the way you recover.

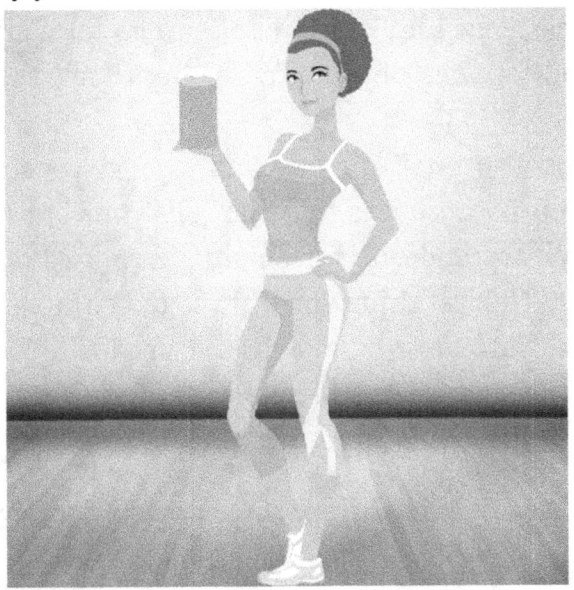

You need to eat or drink about two to three hours before a workout with nutrients that will:

- Sustain your energy
- Boost your performance
- Keep you nicely hydrated
- Preserve your muscle mass
- Speed up your recovery time

Carbohydrates

Carbs are important because consuming these before exercise will fuel your training, giving you lots of energy, and they will also help you recover.

Many people say that you only need carbs if you're going to be engaged in a lengthy workout session, but that's just not true.

Let's say you want to do a shorter workout, but you want it to be high-intensity. You need lots of energy, right?

Unless your idea of exercise is to go for a stroll in the park and feed the birds, you're going to need to stock up on carbs.

Carbs also retain muscle and liver glycogen, which is important because it is this that tells your brain you have been well fed and don't need any more food during your workout. The last thing you want is to get hungry after 30 minutes. Carbs also stimulate the production of insulin, which prevents protein breakdown. Moreover, this is why you absolutely need to start juicing and stop drinking sugary energy drinks.

Fats

Healthy fats are another essential macronutrient that you need.

The funny thing about fats is that they don't improve your performance - but they don't really weaken it either. What they do is slow down digestion, which keeps your body on an even keel in terms of its insulin and blood glucose levels. They also provide you with some micronutrients, too.

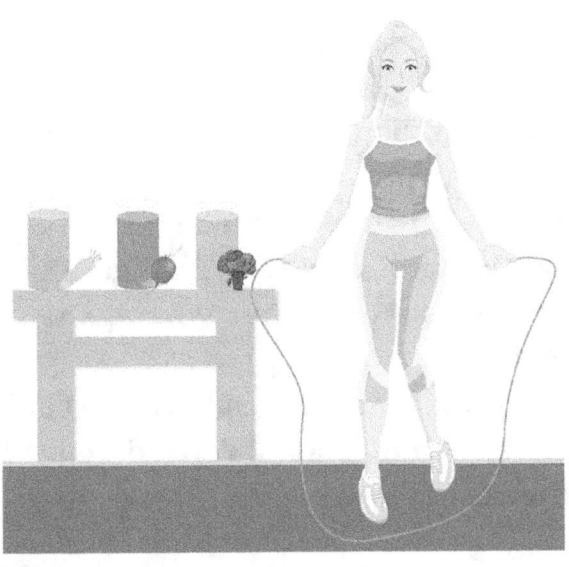

Protein

You can drink some of your juice during exercise, and it should be high protein because protein helps to prevent muscle breakdown, which leads to a better recovery post-workout. It also ensures that you adapt better to training as you progress, which means that you are better able to power your way through your workout.

You don't need a massive amount of protein in your juice; just a small amount is enough to prevent protein breakdown. If you like exercising on an empty stomach, then you don't need any more than around 15 grams of protein during training.

Athletes who do punishing training bouts need more protein, as does anyone who is looking to gain a significant amount of mass.

Micronutrients

Lots of people know how to get their macronutrients - such as fats, carbs and protein - but they don't always stop to think about the role that vitamins and minerals (micronutrients) play in helping them power their way through a workout.

- ✓ **Micronutrients play a really key role in energy production**
- ✓ **They also help to strengthen bones, boost your immune system, instigate hemoglobin synthesis, and protect you against oxidative damage**
- ✓ **Vitamins and minerals also repair muscle tissue that has been damaged during exercise.**

You have to remember that workout stresses numerous metabolic pathways, and if we are to stay on top of these pathways and aid their recovery, we need micronutrients.

It's the same as when a car breaks down on a highway - it needs assistance from an auto repair company, otherwise, it's just dead on its wheels.

Moreover, when we exercise more and more, we experience muscle biochemical adaptations. To cope with these changes, we need even more micronutrients.

Even routine exercise can lead to a loss of too many micronutrients. These leaves you feeling fatigued. It doesn't help you to finish off a workout. Your body takes ages to repair, and you may even come away with a few injuries.

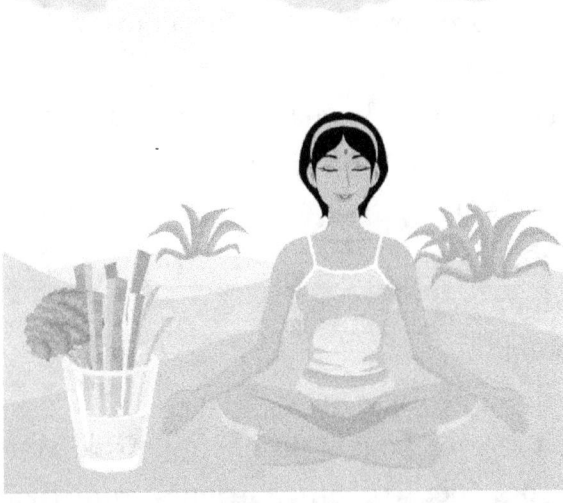

The key nutrients that athletes include in their diets are:

- Calcium
- Vitamin B
- Vitamin C
- Vitamin D
- Vitamin E
- Iron
- Magnesium

And the best place to get more micronutrients? From juicing, of course.

Why?

Juicing is easy, and convenient, what is more convenient than drinking your nutrients?

An 8-ounce vegetable juice blend is like eating 2 large salads without the dressing.

It's portable, so you can easily drink them on your way to the gym, and on the drive home!

Key Nutrients That Power Your Workout
B-Vitamins

If you've been working out for almost an hour but you find yourself running out of steam towards the end, the problem could be that you're lacking in B vitamins.

B Vitamins include:

- Thiamin
- Riboflavin
- Vitamin B-6
- Folate
- Vitamin B-12

If you've ever bought an energy drink, you may have noticed that they contain nutrients from the B-vitamin family, including thiamin, B12, riboflavin, and many others. The reason for this is that B-vitamins give you a burst of energy. They're essential for the conversion of food into fuel. Essential really means essential because without them you will have little energy. The body uses the B-vitamins to convert sugar and protein into fuel so athletes get as many of them as they can.

According to experts from the Department of Nutrition at Arizona State University which posted on MedlinePlus Health Information, B-vitamins, which include thiamin, riboflavin, and vitamin B-6) are necessary for energy-producing pathways in the body. Additionally, folate and vitamin B-12 are necessary to synthesize new red blood cells and to repair damaged cells. Active individuals with a B-vitamin deficit may experience diminished performance during high intensity workouts.

The **major difference between vitamin B from juices made at home and that energy drink** is the latter is filled with other bad ingredients that have landed people in the emergency room, but your juice only has fresh produce and nutrients - **Winning!**

Calcium

You've probably heard all about calcium and how it strengthens the bones and you probably realize that a super strong skeleton is fundamental if you're going to working out, right?

Therefore, it makes sense that calcium should be one of the key nutrients that power your workouts. It increases your bone density, which ensures that your skeleton is strong enough for a great workout.

Milk is not the only source of calcium, you can get it from vegetables, and it's a better source since vegetables have no fat, no cholesterol, and they are low in calories.

Vitamin C

Did you know that if you work out in colder climates, you could suffer from exercise-induced asthma? Not to raise any alarm bells, but that chesty cough you've been battling with these past few months could in fact be asthma.

In addition, it could be that your immune system is not as healthy as you might think. This can be resolved with Vitamin C, which naturally occurs in citrus fruits and various vegetables, and can boost your immunity, protect your cells from free radicals, and a slew of other functions that builds a better body that is powered for exercise.

Moreover, the more vitamin C you have, the easier it is to avoid contracting the flu and the common cold.

Vitamin D

We all need vitamin D, right? Vitamin D comes from the sun and it makes us feel amazing. For many of us, the more sun we have the better we feel. It just imbues us with positivity and motivation. Vitamin D boosts your mood, and in this way, it can increase your determination to make it through a workout like a beast.

However, your mood alone will not get you through all the obstacles; you need something more. You need power, too. You don't need to go searching too far, though, because according to Science Daily vitamin D has been studied and found to be linked with increased muscle efficiency.

It may also be fantastic at tightening up your skeletal muscle function. These are some pretty awesome findings.

Vitamin E

When we're sick, we don't really feel like doing anything. We're just not at our best. We don't feel like filing all those documents at work, going out on that date tonight ... and we especially don't feel in the mood for powering through the workout.

It's funny, but it always seems as though some people are more susceptible to getting sick than others are. Perhaps it's you that always seems to be sick, while your friends are constantly motoring through their work out like a warrior.

The reason for this could be that you are deficient in vitamin E. Consuming more vitamin E can lower your risk of infection. It can make you almost immune to the common cold, the flu, and can slash your risk of developing pneumonia by almost 70%.

Iron

Popeye loved his spinach because he knew it contained lots of iron that would power his way through a workout. His nemesis Bluto must have loved the dark leafy green even more, because he was even bigger!

Iron is one of the key nutrients you need a lot more of if you want to own your workouts and fight fatigue; it's also integral in the metabolizing proteins, hemoglobin production, and red blood cell health.

Here is some quick science:

- Each time you work out for an hour, your body loses around 5.6% of iron. That's quite significant.
- What happens next is your red blood cells struggle to carry as much oxygen to your muscles.
- Moreover, when your muscles don't get enough oxygen, you quickly get fatigued and may not be able to complete your workout.

Magnesium

Magnesium is an absolute powerhouse mineral that top athletes make a priority. Magnesium is actually composed of over 300 enzymes that aid energy metabolism.

It also helps to strengthen your bones, which as previously mentioned is vital for your workout. As well as having a strong skeleton, you always need to avoid stress fractures as much as possible, and magnesium will help you do just that.

In addition, because you lose a lot of magnesium through sweat, you really need to consume as much of it as possible to replenish the supply lost in your workouts.

Potassium

No doubt, you've seen tennis players munching away on bananas during a break in play. This is because bananas are super rich in potassium, a vital nutrient that speeds up recovery and nips cramps in the bud.

Juicing for Micronutrients: Key Ingredients

Now that you know that what key micronutrients you need to power your workout, you're probably wondering about the best sources for these, here are your best fruit and vegetable sources that will provide you with much needed nutrition through power juicing.

Calcium

Calcium is found in quite a few great juicing vegetables, which means that you get to choose what works for you.

- **Kale** is incredibly rich in calcium, and is one of the most popular juicing vegetables, making up the bulk of the very healthy green juice. It delivers 139mg of calcium per every 100g serving. The best thing is that it's easily absorbed by the body.
- **Broccoli** is another great vegetable for juicing that is a fantastic source of calcium, and a single cup serving returns around 74mg.
- **Spinach** is a good leafy green alternative to kale (or you can juice both together), that contains around 145mg of calcium for every 100g serving. Yes, that's even better than kale.
- **Kelp** is also another fantastic source of calcium; a single cup serving returns around 136mg of this essential nutrient.

Vitamin C

Vitamin C could easily turn out to be your favorite micronutrient because so many tasty fruits and vegetables are loaded with it.

- The exotic and super delicious **guavas** always add a kick to juices, and a 100g serving contains a whopping 228mg of vitamin C.
- **Kiwifruit** might be something of an acquired taste, but if you love it, you're going to love the fact that a 100g serving contains 92mg of vitamin C.
- **Strawberries** are also rich in vitamin C, with a 100g serving containing almost 60mg of the nutrient.
- Then there are the zesty **citrus fruits**, ideal for juicing and specially to enhance the flavor of vegetable juices. **Lemons, limes, grapefruits** give you around 53mg of vitamin C per fruit.
- **Apples** contain lots of vitamin C, as do **tomatoes, kale,** and **broccoli.**

Vitamin E

- **Avocados** don't juice well, however they can be blended and mixed in with juice for a half and half smoothie juice blend. A 100g serving is enough to return 2.2mg of the often hard-to-get-hold-of vitamin E.
- **Sunflower seeds are loaded with vitamin E,** 36mg for every 100g serving and they are a great source of healthy fats. You can sprinkle these on top of your juice or grind them up and stir into a ready-made juice.

- **Broccoli** is also a good source of vitamin E, with a 100g serving delivering 1.5mg to your body and broccoli juices great.

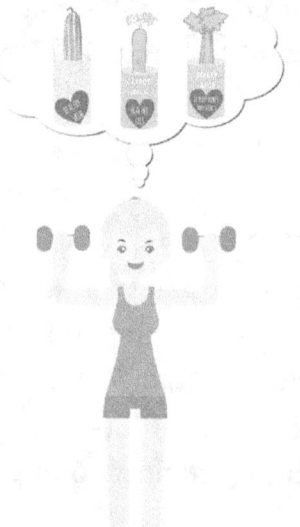

- **Squash** and **pumpkin** return around 1.3mg each per 100g serving, while **blackberries** are 8% vitamin E, **peaches** are 7%, and **raspberries** are 5%.

Iron

- You can look to **spinach** for your iron intake. This dark leafy green vegetable delivers 3.57mg of iron per ever 100g serving.
- **Asparagus** is another good source, and returns 2.14mg of iron for every 100g serving.
- Berries are really good sources, too: **elderberries** are 13% iron, while **raspberries** are 9% and **blackberries** are 5%.
- If you want to try something a little bit different in your juice, how about **coconut**? A 100g serving contains 3.32mg of iron.

Potassium

Many fruits and vegetables are rich in potassium.

- **Guavas**, which contain 417mg per 100g serving.
- **Bananas** are well known for their potassium content, and they return 358mg per 100g serving.

Bananas don't juice, but they blend so you can stir them into your finished juices.

- **Spinach** juices great and has 167mg per I cup, if you juice 3 cups you are getting more than 15% of the daily recommended value of potassium.
- **Passion fruit** should be on your grocery list too, as this silky fruit contains 348mg per 100g serving.
- **Apricots** are also a good source of potassium, with every 100g serving returning 259mg.
- **Pomegranates** contain 236mg per 100g serving, while **cherries** deliver 222mg to your body.

Magnesium

- All dark leafy greens, including **Kale, spinach, chard, and collard greens** are high in magnesium.
- **Cherries, coconut, papaya, bananas, watermelon, and peaches** are your best fruit choices for magnesium intake.

Vitamin D

There are many choices in great juicing fruits and vegetables for vitamin D.

- **Kale** is one of the best sources of vitamin D supplying 6,693 IU per cup
- **Spinach** comes in second with 2,813 IU per cup
- **Swiss chard** has 2,202 IU per cup
- You can also get it from, **kohlrabi, asparagus, bitter melon** including the leafy tops, **broccoli, cauliflower, zucchini** and **cucumber**
- **Grapefruits** with 2,830 IU per fruit
- **Mangoes** 1,785 IU per 1 cup

- **Papaya** with 1,492 IU per 1 small fruit
- **Tomatoes**, with 1,025 IU per 1 medium tomato
- **Watermelon** has 865 IU per 1 cup diced
- Other fruits include, **cranberries, gooseberries, grapes, passionfruit, and peaches**

B-Vitamins

Riboflavin

Vegetable sources include **beet Greens, Asparagus, spinach, collard greens, Dandelion Greens** and other **dark green leafy vegetables, peppers, Brussels sprouts, Asparagus** and **Broccoli.**

Fresh fruit sources include **blueberries, apples, passion fruit,** and **avocado.** When it comes to fruit, many offer higher counts in dried form which is not appropriate for juicing, plus dried fruit is not your best choice in any case, since it is much higher in sugar than fresh fruit.

Folate

Vegetable sources include **leafy greens** such as **spinach** and **turnip greens**

Fruit sources include **oranges** with the most at about 50 mcg per fruit and one large glass of orange juice providing even more. Other folate-rich fruits include **grapes, banana, cantaloupe, papaya, grapefruit,** and **strawberries**.

Vitamin B6

Vegetable sources include leafy green vegetables: **spinach, kale, greens,** and **broccoli.**

Fruit sources include **bananas.**

The Power of Beets

This chapter is dedicated to beets, which can go a long way to power your workouts and improve your overall performance.

Beets Contain a Wealth of Nutrients

Yes, beets contain a wide variety of healthy nutrients, including:

- Beets are a unique source of phytonutrients called betalains that have anti- antioxidant, anti-inflammatory, and detoxification properties.
- Beetroots are rich in inorganic nitrates, which are compounds that encourage the signaling molecule Nitric Oxide to take action.
- Folate - 34% DRI/DV per 1 cup
- Manganese - 28% DRI/DV per 1 cup
- Potassium - 15% DRI/DV per 1 cup
- Copper - 14% DRI/DV per 1 cup
- Fiber - 14% DRI/DV per 1 cup
- Magnesium - 10% DRI/DV per 1 cup
- Phosphorus - 9% DRI/DV per 1 cup
- Vitamin C - 8% DRI/DV per 1 cup
- Iron - 7% DRI/DV per 1 cup
- Vitamin B6 - 6% DRI/DV per 1 cup

Benefits

✓ Beetroots are so good for you as they improve brain functioning, which is what you need when the

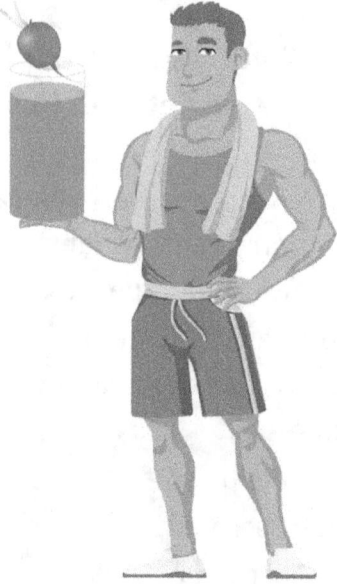

tough gets going down at the gym. Many people underestimate the power of mental resilience, but you should never underestimate it.

✓ Beets also promote stronger bones, and as we all know a super strong skeleton is essential for a good workout.

✓ Beets also boost your immune system lowering your chances of getting sick and missing days at the gym.

Yet people keep on ignoring these purple veggies whenever they do their weekly shop. As a matter of fact, beetroots must be one of the most overlooked veggies in America. It's amazing how people who see these colorful vegetables screaming at them "pick me! pick me!" but opt for lettuce again, as usual.

Get out of your comfort zone, and get into juicing beetroots. Elite athletes all around the world use them, and they'll tell you that beets are the vegetables that give them the edge over their competitors.

The Science Behind Beets

Beetroots are rich in inorganic nitrates, which are compounds that encourage the signaling molecule Nitric Oxide to take action.

NO is made in our bodies but we don't always produce very much of it. To produce more of it, we need to eat food that is rich in nitrate - such as beets.

NO improves the strength of our skeleton, and increases the amount of oxygen that is sent to our brain.

Why Juice Beets?

According to research, drinking around 500ml of beetroot juice per day can keep us feeling more energetic. In fact, drinking beet juice can keep us going in the gym for 15% more time than we normally would.

Many people think that juicing just takes up too much time, and it's too messy. However, when you have the right equipment and plan ahead, it is much easier than you think.

If you have the time to make yourself some juice in the morning before a workout, this is something you should definitely think about doing.

Alternatives include beet powder and concentrated juices, but these are often filled with artificial substances, too much sugar, and not enough fiber or nutrients - basically, they don't have the same amount of good stuff as beet juice does.

How Much Do You Need?

As previously stated, 500ml of beet juice per day is enough to increase our staying power by around 15%. This equates to 2 cups. However, go ahead find a dose that works for you, if 250ml of beet juice a day increases you're staying power by 10%, then go for it.

Some athletes drink more than 600ml, but again it's all about how much you can handle.

Cooked or Raw

Research in the past has shown that cooking beetroots can reduce the nitrates content - which is not what we really want. For this reason, it's best to juice with raw beets only.

Drink It Slow

It takes a while for the nitrates in beets to be ingested, and used by your body. They enter our mouth, where they are manipulated by saliva. This takes a bit of time, so if you clean your teeth not long after eating (and many people do this after eating beets in order to get rid of the purple color) you will only be washing all the beneficial nitrates out of your mouth. Drink slowly for better conversion rates.

Does It Work for Everyone?

Beet juice works for many people, many boost their workouts, but like with anything, our body's all respond in different ways. What works for some might not work for others. The only really accurate way you can find out is by giving it a go. Other high nitrate vegetables include spinach and kale.

Juicing for Better Aging

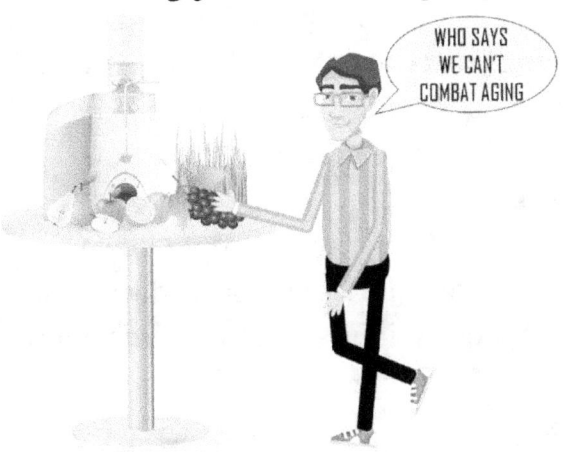

WHO SAYS WE CAN'T COMBAT AGING

Combat Aging with Juicing

While you can reduce the signs of aging by eating plenty of vegetables and fruits, not everyone can tolerate large amounts of fruits and vegetables in their daily diet. This is where juicing comes it.

Juicing involves putting vegetables and fruits through a juicer, where the produce is ground into a healthy juice that you can drink to achieve the benefits of the nutrients.

Juicing is a good way to get your fruits and vegetables. While it removes the insoluble fiber, it keeps the soluble fiber, which is important in its own right.

An 8 oz. glass of green juice is like eating 2 large salads without dressing!

You can increase the body's absorption of key phytonutrients when you get the insoluble fiber out of the way. The healthy enzymes in juice will be able to be absorbed better without the insoluble fiber. If you have a hard time eating whole vegetables, then juicing is the right option for you.

While juicing is certainly not a miracle cure for disease, nor can it stop the aging process, it is certainly a great arm of defense against the effects of aging because solid nutrition is still one of the best ways to prevent disease, and boost health and wellness.

General Health

Juicing green vegetables breaks down their cell walls making their key nutrients easy to digest allowing you to quickly and easily infuse your body with phytonutrients, enzymes, oxygen, chlorophyll, vitamins, antioxidants, and minerals.

Nutrition plays a key role in how well we age, or whether we wind up dealing with disease and consequent premature death.

The top cause of death in the United States and other countries around the world is heart disease. According to the Centers for Disease Control, a majority of heart disease is preventable as is it attributed to lifestyle choices, like diet and exercise.

When the body gets proper nutrition, the immune system remains healthy, as do many of the vital internal body process that play a key role in your health and wellness.

Age Fighting Antioxidants

Juicing will provide you with age-fighting antioxidants. Antioxidants are molecules that scavenge for oxygen free radicals that are missing an electron and are looking for any molecule of the cell to give it to them, including the DNA.

By protecting DNA, antioxidants can be preventative against cancerous mutations that can occur in the DNA.

The antioxidants in juices can prevent cell death, which makes it a good choice to fight the aging process.

As we get older, it gets harder and harder to maintain good health. From stress at work to the temptation of fast food and harmful exposure to pollution and UV rays, there are countless factors that can make the privilege of aging a difficult, and painful, process.

However, when you incorporate foods rich in antioxidants into your diet, you can actually undo the effects of aging and earn back the health of youth.

Even more, increasing your antioxidant levels when you're young can not only slow the aging process, but also help you stay healthier for much longer. Below are some of the amazing ways that antioxidants can improve the aging process for years to come.

Improving and Protecting the Skin

The state of your skin carries the biggest visual link to aging, as nearly everyone associates wrinkles and splotches with getting old. Instead of paying a fortune for expensive serums and plastic surgery, you can keep your skin smooth and taught by maintaining a diet high in antioxidants.

Antioxidants help your skin maintain its elasticity by preserving the strength of collagen, the tissue that makes up your skin. Free radicals break down collagen over time, which causes it to sag, droop, and even develop uneven coloring. Keeping your skin strong and healthy also reduces the chances of developing skin conditions and can even fight off skin cancer, commonly associated with long-term exposure to UV rays.

Juicing is good for your skin. Choose vegetables that have vitamins in them that increase the production of collagen. You need collagen to fill out your tissues and decrease the chances of having wrinkles.

Collagen-producing vegetables and fruits include:
- Cabbage
- Any Red Fruit or Vegetable
- Carrots
- Flaxseeds (can be ground and stirred into your juice)

Hemp seeds help improve the radiance and firmness of skin and they are the only edible source of linoleic acid (GLA) that provides omega-6 fatty acids that are part of the membrane around skin cells. This protein rich plant food helps synthesize collagen and elastin to improve skin firmness and keep it looking supple. Ground hemp seeds can be easily added to juices and smoothies.

Reducing Memory Loss

One of the hardest parts about getting older is struggling with memory loss. Whether it's a general forgetfulness that makes it hard to find your keys in the morning or more serious issues in the form of diseases such as Alzheimer's, everyone experiences it differently.

Fortunately, everyone can improve their memory and fight off these cognitive impairments with antioxidants. These nutrients help to undue damage to the brain and remove senile plaque in the grey matter of the brain, which makes it harder for it to function. They also improve your recall ability by increasing your mental agility and giving you more energy to carry out higher brain functions.

Promoting A Healthy Heart

The heart experiences high levels of wear over the years, which can result in an increased likelihood of a heart attack as you age. Antioxidants keep your heart strong by reducing the damage caused by free radicals, which can appear during fat oxidation throughout the body. As these free radicals build up, they damage the walls of the heart and blood vessels, which can literally weaken the hart and decrease its ability to function.

They also make the heart more susceptible to the buildup of harmful cholesterols. Over time, cholesterol deposits in the heart can create blockages that decrease blood flow. This can force the heart to work harder, which can result in a heart attack, as well as limit the amount of blood that travels through the body and cause widespread damage.

Increasing Resilience to Disease

Antioxidants can help to strengthen your immune system in a variety of ways, which can help with everything from fighting off a common cold to protecting you from the development of cancer. One key function of the immune system is to block the passage of harmful compounds throughout the body through inflammation.

A weak immune system is not able to prevent these compounds from spreading, while a damaged one may over inflame and lead to other major complications.

Antioxidants and flavonoids in particular, keep your immune system in check and help it to fight off diseases.

They also reduce the likelihood of developing diabetes, suffering from a stroke and the onset of arthritis, all of which become more prominent and harmful with age.

Additionally, several studies have shown promise in the spice turmeric reducing risks for cancer, and it makes a great addition to various juice blends.

Fruits and Vegetables Rich in Antioxidants

Berries are some of the best sources and they are also low in sugar.

- Wild blueberries have 13,427 per 1 cup
- Blueberries (cultivated) have 9,019 per 1 cup
- Cranberries have 8,983 per 1 cup
- Blackberries have 7,701 per 1 cup
- Raspberries have 6,058 per 1 cup
- Strawberries have 5,938 per 1 cup

Specific Antioxidants and Their Sources

- **Allium sulphur compounds:** Leeks and garlic
- **Anthocyanins:** Eggplant, grapes, and all berries
- **Beta carotene:** apricots, carrots, spinach, pumpkin, mangoes and parsley
- **Cryptoxanthins:** Red peppers, pumpkin and mangoes
- **Flavonoids:** Citrus fruits and apples
- **Indoles:** Cruciferous vegetable varieties, including leafy greens, broccoli, cabbage, and cauliflower
- **Lignans:** Broccoli, curly kale, Brussels sprouts, cauliflower, white and red cabbage, carrots, green and red sweet peppers.

- **Lutein:** All leafy greens, including, collards, Swiss chard, kale and spinach
- **Lycopene:** Tomatoes have the highest content plus it's found in pink grapefruit and watermelon
- **Polyphenols:** Thyme and oregano
- **Vitamin C:** Oranges, mangoes, broccoli, spinach, berries, kiwi fruit and peppers
- **Vitamin E:** Avocados

Weight loss as we indicated before juicing can help with weight loss. Instead of a large fatty meal, you can juice up some fresh fruits and vegetables that are naturally low in calories.

The Connection Between Obesity and Aging

The term obesity doesn't tie exclusively into a specific weight or body fat percentage, which can lead many people to be in denial about their condition. The best way to approach the matter is with honesty, understanding that hiding from

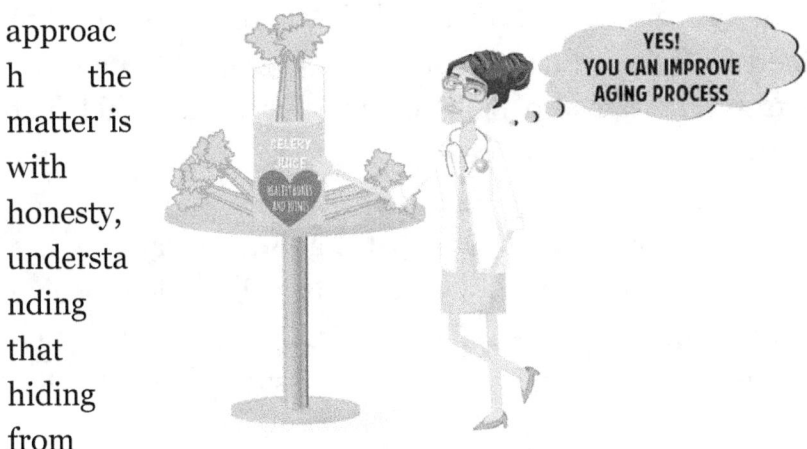

excess body fat is literally shaving years off your life.

Being overweight is something everybody struggles with as they age because the metabolism naturally slows down over time, meaning that it becomes less effective at converting food into energy.

For many, joint pains and other body aches—as well as a generally sedentary lifestyle, such as working in an office—can also lead to a decrease in physical activity and in turn a lower calorie burn. Over time, this kind of lifestyle taxes the body and leaves it much weaker and more susceptible to illness.

Increased Risk Across the Board

The major issue is that obesity worsens the effects of other ailments that occur during aging. For example, being overweight puts more strain on your heart because it has to work harder to move your now heavier body.

As excess body fat often comes as a result of a poor diet, this also means that high levels of cholesterol are more likely and thus you are more susceptible to a heart attack. Fat can also build up in your lungs, making it harder for you to breathe and leading to a faster deterioration of your muscles.

Other issues, such as diabetes and joint damage, are also made worse by obesity, which is bad for older people because the body just can't recover like it used to, which makes every sickness and every issue potentially life threatening.

Fighting Back with Juicing

Juicing fresh fruits and vegetables is one of the best ways to battle obesity, especially when age is an issue, because it can give your body the boost it needs to undo all the damage. For example, a juice cleanse routine that combines leafy greens such as kale and cabbage with high-fiber vegetables such as carrots and antioxidant-rich blueberries can clear out many of the harmful chemicals and compounds that build up over time.

A diet of highly processed foods and red meats can cause constipation, liver failure, and excess plaque in the blood vessels. The vitamins and minerals in these foods give your body the nutrients it needs flush the bad stuff out and start repairing itself.

While there is nothing more effective for weight loss than regular exercise, adding fresh fruit and vegetable juice to your routine can also have a major impact. Apples, spinach, berries, and cucumbers can help you feel more satiated throughout the day.

When you feel full, it's much easier to fight the cravings and temptations and stick to a healthy diet. They also carry huge levels of antioxidants, vitamins, and proteins that your body needs to repair muscles, increase your energy levels and even help you burn more calories during your workouts.

Energy

Juices can give you extra energy from the antioxidants in cruciferous vegetables and berries, along with beets and carrots, which are high in phytonutrients.

From the moment you wake up until you're finally settling into bed, staying energized can be a struggle. If you're like most people, you turn to caffeine, sugar, and energy drinks to stay awake and keep functioning, and you probably do it excessively often.

A dependence on these sources, natural or artificial, can not only lead to some serious medical issues, but also actually make you more tired overall.

Boost Brain Health

Juicing can boost your memory and cognitive abilities.

However, you might not know that you can tailor your juicing to give you a significant boost in brain health. Just like all the other organs in the body, the brain experiences wear, as we get older, which means it starts to function less efficiently and becomes more susceptible to disease.

If you want to make sure your mind is in tiptop shape, read on to learn about the basics of brain health and what ingredients you can juice to keep it strong.

What Makes a Healthy Brain?

The brain is arguably the most important component in the body, controlling everything we do, think and feel. However, you can't work it out like other muscles. This means that the only way you can keep your brain healthy is be targeting it with nutrients such as Vitamin E, lycopene, antioxidants, Zinc and essential fatty acids.

When you work these essential vitamins and minerals into your diet, you can help stave off the effects of diseases such as dementia, fight memory loss, and reversing cognitive impairments. They can also help you to think more quickly, maintain focus and give you the energy to tackle more complex problems. Think of them like a fuel additive in a car, clearing out build up and giving it an extra boost in performance.

The Power of the Blue Berry

One of the most effective foods to increase your brain health is **blueberries**. These superfoods are jam packed with antioxidants, which are good for your whole body as well as your brain. Several studies have linked the antioxidants in blueberries with a decrease in oxidative stress to the brain, linked to diseases such as Alzheimer's, as well as an increase in the ability to learn new skills, according to WebMD.com.

Other Colorful Fruits and Vegetables

Other dark berries, such as **blackberries, raspberries** and also **cherries** have high levels of flavonoids that have a positive impact on your memory overall.

Also, look to those fruits you often think of as vegetables, such as **tomatoes** and **avocados**, for huge doses of other types of antioxidants and healthy fats to boost these results.

Veggies That Pack a Smart Punch

If you're looking for some greens to add to your brain-boosting juices, stick to the cruciferous family.

Foods such as **broccoli, kale** and other **dark leafy greens** are essential for memory. These foods are full of Vitamin K, which helps to improve your recall abilities and strengthens your memory overall.

Juicing **spinach** can also give you iron, which not only promotes the creation of hemoglobin, which is vital to your body's repairing process, but Zinc as well. Zinc does a lot of good for your body, and specifically boosts your thinking ability by helping your brain better utilize the synapses.

Turmeric protects brain cells from free radical damage to improve concentration and fresh turmeric can be juiced along with other vegetables.

Adding Seeds for an Extra Boost

Take your juicing to the next level of brain health by working in ground seeds, which offer amazingly high levels of all the best nutrients without increasing the total calorie count.

A tablespoon of **flaxseed** can give you a huge dose of Omega-3 fatty acids, which can decrease the effects of cognitive impairments and memory loss associated with aging.

Pumpkin seeds are also a great source of zinc, and can add a seasonal flavor to your juices. In order to get the biggest benefit, focus on seeds with a high concentration of docosahexaenoic acid.

This essential fatty acid is found in large quantities in the brain during youth, so keeping your levels high helps your brain to function at a younger level and combat other age-related memory issues.

Juicing for Cancer

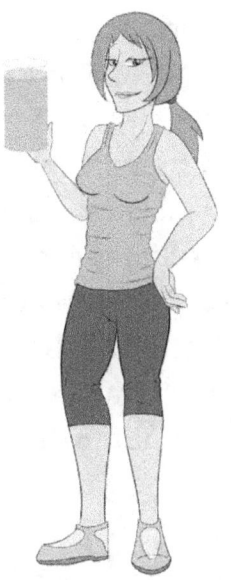

Best Juicing Vegetables There are several raw vegetables that are especially recommended for reducing risks for various types of cancer. Many also utilize these vegetables as a support in fighting cancer once a diagnosis has been made.

Of course, no scientific evidence exists that juicing or eating these vegetables can cure cancer, or guarantee that you will never get it, but it is true that healthy nutrient rich juices can boost immunity, promote energy, which is often drained during cancer treatments and boost your overall health.

Furthermore, scientific research has found promising results in certain vegetables playing a key role in cancer prevention.

Cruciferous Vegetables

Cruciferous vegetables are part of the Brassica genus plant family. These vegetables are rich in key nutrients, including carotenoids, such as lutein, beta-carotene, and zeaxanthin. They are also rich sources of key vitamins, including vitamins C, E, and K along with folate and minerals.

Moreover, these gems of nature provide a group of substances known as glucosinolates, which are chemicals that contain sulfur. It is the sulfur that gives some of these vegetables their bitter flavor, like that in greens.

According to the National Cancer Institute, animal studies and lab grown cell experiments have identified numerous potential ways in which glucosinolates can help in preventing cancer:

- Protect cells from DNA damage
- Ability to inactivate carcinogens
- Hold antiviral, anti-inflammatory and antibacterial properties
- Induce apoptosis or cell death
- Hinder tumor blood vessel formation and migration, which is required for metastasis

The following section details some of the cruciferous vegetables that are best for juicing.

Broccoli

Broccoli contains high levels of sulforaphane, a very potent compound that increases the body's protective enzymes and flushes out cancer-causing chemicals. Juice the whole vegetable, including the stems, leaves, and florets as they hold key nutrients.

Cabbage

Another member of the cruciferous family of vegetables that provides powerful antioxidants including, vitamins A and C and the phytonutrients, zeaxanthin, isothiocyanates, thiocyanates, lutein, and sulforaphane that stimulate detoxifying enzymes, fight oxidative stress and may offer protection from prostate, colon, and even breast cancers.

In addition, sulforaphane selectively targets cancer stem cells that may prevent cancer from spreading or even recurring.

Cabbage juice is probably not the tastiest on its own, but can be added to delicious cancer fighting blends that include, kale, green apples, berries, and beets.

Kale

According to the National Cancer Institute, kale is yet another valuable cruciferous vegetable that has promise in helping humans will the battle against cancer.

Kale is rich in important nutrients, such as lutein, zeaxanthin, vitamins C, E, and K; folate; and minerals. Kale also contains glucosinolates, or sulfur-containing chemicals. While the folate found in kale does not have a direct impact on cancer treatment, it does help to reduce the risk of complications from cancer and its treatment by lowering risks for heart disease.

Kale and beets are rich sources of potassium, which is an electrolyte that helps regulate fluid in the body, move nutrients into the cells, and remove waste from cells, and supports the communication between nerves and muscles.

While potassium does not have a direct effect on preventing cancer, it may be beneficial depending upon medications that are prescribed during cancer treatment and side effects that result from treatment, ask your doctor.

While human studies have shown mixed results, it is 100% safe to say that kale is a nutrient rich plant food that is 100% recommended as part of a daily balanced diet and should the cancer fighting promise materialize that is just icing on the cake.

Kale juices great, and blends wonderfully with many different nutritious fruits and vegetables. It may be an acquired taste for some, but adding lemon or lime juice, and a green apple to kale makes it very tasty.

Other Cruciferous Vegetables:
- Arugula
- Bok Choy
- Brussels Sprouts
- Collard Greens
- Radishes
- Rutabaga
- Turnips
- Watercress

Carrots

Carrots contain natural compounds, poly-acetylenes that are only found in carrots and ginseng and that protect the plant from pests and disease.

Various tests have shown poly-acetylenes to fight inflammation and cancer and reduce cancer growth in rats. Carrots also contain beta-carotene, alpha carotene, vitamin E, and other cancer fighting nutrients.

Carrots are higher in sugar than green vegetables, so watch your juicing intake. Carrot juice blends great with kale, cabbage, and green apples.

Beets

These colorful purple gems of nature contain betacyanin that researchers believe could protect against the development of cancer cells, and may possibly reduce risks for inflammation, which promotes malignancy.

Beets are wonderful for juicing and a great blend is 3 small beets, 1 cucumber, 1 handful of spinach and an orange.

Turmeric

Turmeric is not technically a vegetable, but a spice that is often used in Asian and Indian cooking and belongs to the ginger family. It is grown in Asian countries and has been used for centuries in herbal medicine.

Turmeric contains curcumin that is believed by experts to have exceptional anti-inflammatory abilities, which makes it effective for fighting cancer because most diseases are caused by and thrive under a state of chronic and long-term inflammation, according to a biochemist at The University of Texas M. D. Anderson Cancer Center, Bharat B. Aggarwal, PhD. Recent studies found curcumin to interfere with cell-signaling pathways that suppress the transformation, proliferation, and invasion of cancer cells.

According to Cancer Research UK, curcumin was found to stop pre-cancerous changes to becoming cancer when given to 25 patients with pre-cancerous changes in different organs in a phase 1 clinical trial.

Analytical research has found that certain type of cancer rates are lowest in countries where curcumin is consumed at levels of about 100 to 200 mg a day regularly.

Numerous lab studies on cancer cells have found curcumin to have anticancer effects, as it not only killed cancer cells but also prevented their growth. These studies found these effects to be most profound on skin, bowel, breast, and stomach cancer cells.

A 2007 study done in the United States, found that a combination of curcumin and chemotherapy killed more bowel cancer cells than chemotherapy alone. Another 2007 US study of mice found that curcumin helped to stop the spread of breast cancer cells to other parts of the body.

How to Use in Juicing

Fresh turmeric can be juiced along with other fruits and vegetables. Another option is to add 1 or 2 teaspoons of the ground spice into your juices and enjoy the health boost!

Garlic

The phytochemicals found in garlic help to stop the formation of nitrosamines, which are carcinogens formed in the stomach, and under certain conditions in the intestines.

Garlic is a vegetable that's part of the Allium class of bulb-shaped plants that also features leeks, onions, chives, and scallions.

Garlic contains an unusually high amount of sulfur along with flavonoids, arginine, oligosaccharides, and selenium.

Garlic's pungent odor and flavor stems from the sulfur compounds, which are formed from allicin, a major precursor of the bioactive compounds in garlic formed when garlic cloves are crushed or chopped.

These bioactive compounds are defined as elements in food other than those needed for basic nutrition, but are responsible for changes in health.

According to the National Cancer Institute, several multidisciplinary studies of population groups that investigate causes, spread of, incidence and effect of certain health-related interventions, nutritional intakes, or environmental exposures, have shown a relationship between increases in intake of garlic and a reduction in risks for cancers of the pancreas, breast, stomach, colorectal, esophagus and colon.

The Iowa Women's Study is looked into whether diet, body fat distribution along with other risk factors contribute to cancer rates in older women. The study has found that women who eat the highest amounts of garlic reduced their risk for colon cancer by 50% cancer as compared to women whose consumption levels were much lower (Steinmetz KA et al, American Journal of Epidemiology 1994; 139(1):1–15.).

Higher intakes of onion and garlic were associated with a reduced risk of intestinal cancer in the European Prospective Investigation into Cancer and Nutrition, which involves men and women from 10 different countries (Gonzalez CA, Pera G, Agudo A, et al.).

Numerous population studies conducted in China that centered on intake of garlic and cancer risk have found a strong connection between garlic and lower cancer rates.

One of these studies, found that regular and frequent intake of garlic reduced risk for esophageal and stomach cancers and risk factors grew with higher consumption levels (Gao, Takezaki, Ding, Li, Tajima, et al).

Another one of the studies in China found that high intake of garlic and onions reduced risk for stomach cancer (Setiawan VW, et al).

Yet another study found that the greater the intake of garlic and scallions, meaning more than 10 grams daily versus less than 2.2 grams per day was associated with about a 50% reduction in prostate cancer risk (Hsing AW et al).

A study in France found that higher intake of garlic was linked with a statistically significant reduction in risk for breast cancer.

A study conducted in the San Francisco Bay area (Chan JM, Wang F, Holly EA.) discovered a 54% lower risk for pancreatic cancer in people who had a high intake of garlic versus those who ate much less.

How to Use in Juicing

Juiced garlic is very potent, but just a little bit is all you need, with 1 to 2 cloves added to any of the other vegetables mentioned, and even fruits, like green apples or tomatoes. The other ingredients will mask the pungent flavor allowing you to get your pure raw garlic nutrition without sacrificing taste.

A nice savory juice includes, garlic, tomatoes, cabbage, celery or zucchini, shallots or any onion and red peppers, makes for a great meatless lunch or dinner.

Of course, if you can stand it, go ahead and a get a shot of straight garlic juice daily! Besides cancer, it will help you fight the cold, flu, allergies, sinusitis along with various other respiratory disorders, and it has significant cardiovascular benefits due to its natural ability to reduce vascular inflammation and blood clotting.

Ginger

According to WebMd, researchers have found ginger able to kill cancer cells in two ways.

- In a process called apoptosis, cancer cells kill themselves without harming surrounding healthy cells.
- In another process known as autophagy, cancer cells are duped into digesting themselves as described by J. Rebecca Liu, an assistant professor of obstetrics and gynecology at the University of Michigan doing extensive research on ginger's effects on ovarian cancer cells.

While only preliminary, and animal and human trials are still needed, the research is promising because patient's with ovarian cancer develop resistance to chemotherapy drugs, so ginger's ability to kill cancer cells in more than one way may prove useful.

The Comprehensive Cancer Center at the University of Michigan Health system does not recommend ginger supplements, but does recommend fresh ginger in dietary form not only for its potential cancer fighting role, but also because it is healthy in other ways and works great for nausea.

How to Use in Juicing

Ginger adds a fresh, floral, and crisp flavor to a variety of juice blends, or if you really love it, you can take a small shot of it on its own.

Peel a small piece of fresh ginger with a spoon and add to your juicer, typically a 1" inch piece is more than enough. While ginger does not produce a lot of juice, it does add a lot of flavor so a little goes a long way.

Caution: Avoid excessive amounts if you take blood-thinners or diabetes medication, ask your doctor.

Best Juicing Fruits

Fruit juices can also prevent cancer or even help fight cancer once a diagnosis is made. The American Institute for Cancer Research recommends the following raw fruits to aid in the fight against cancer.

Purple Grapes

Both grapes and juice of grapes including the skin are excellent sources of resveratrol, which is a phytochemical from a group of phytochemicals known as polyphenols.

Numerous studies have suggested that polyphenols and especially resveratrol is a powerful antioxidant that in lab studies has prevented particular damage known to trigger the cancer process in tissues, cells, and animal models.

How to Use in Juicing

Make sure to juice the whole grape, as the skin holds much of the resveratrol. Blend with vegetables for a powerful healthy juice.

Blueberries

Contain cancer fighting phytochemicals, ellagic acid, and anthocyanins. The Institute reports that cell studies of these compounds showed these nutrients to decrease the growth of cancer cells and also to stimulate self-destruction of breast, prostate, mouth, and, colon cancer cells. Centrifugal juicers cannot juice berries and grapes, but masticating and singer-auger juicers can.

How to Use in Juicing

To use blueberries, it is best to blend them, then strain over a bowl with a spout (for easier pouring) to remove the pulp, or better yet leave the pulp and pour the juice and pulp into your main juice, like a blend of kale and other greens. This results in a type of smoothie juice blend.

Watermelon

Watermelon has loads of lycopene, one of the more potent antioxidant shown in research to protect against prostate cancer.

Watermelon is also one of the best fruits for weight control as it really satisfies the sweet tooth with just 49 calories per 2 cup serving.

Since it is one of the lower sugar fruits, it is ideal for juicing and juices quite well.

How to Use in Juicing

Juicing watermelon depends on your juicer model; check the manual to see how much prep is required, for example if the skin should be removed.

Peaches

The peach gets is bright orange color from beta-carotene that helps to reduce inflammation, protect DNA, boost immunity function and plays a key role in controlling cell growth in a way that reduces risks for cancer.

Strawberries

Strawberries contain ellagic acid, a key phytochemical in decreasing growth of cancer cells and stimulating soft-

destruction of cancer cells, such as those in the breast, colon, prostate and mouth.

Furthermore, studies have shown that ellagic acid uses several different cancer-fighting methods simultaneously, as it acts as an antioxidant, slows reproduction of cancer cells, and supports the body in deactivating specific carcinogens.

How to Use in Juicing

Strawberries are more difficult to juice, depending on the model of your juicer. If you have a smoothie maker you can use that or mash them up and add them in after your main juice is ready; this also allows you to get more fiber intake from these healthy berries. A food processor or blender works great too. Strawberries go great with a kale, broccoli, and spinach or any greens.

Apples

Apples contain potent phytochemicals that protect cells from cancer-inducing oxidative damage.

According to the American Institute for Cancer Research, apples can help prevent the start of cancer growth, stop continued tumor growth, and promote cancer cell death.

Laboratory studies conducted by Dr. Rui Hai Liu showed the phytochemicals in apples to suppress breast cancer tumor growth.

The Institute recommends eating one or more apples per day as it is associated with lower risks for both colon and lung cancer in numerous large-scale human studies that evaluated apple consumption and cancer incidence.

How to Use in Juicing

Apples juice great and are a fantastic complimentary flavor to many vegetables. Check your juicer's manual on necessary prep required as they do vary, for example, some allow you to add a whole apple down the feed chute, while others require cutting.

Choose green apples, as they are lowest in sugar.

Tomatoes

One of the best dietary sources of lycopene, a carotenoid that plays a key role in cancer prevention and was found to stop endometrial cancer (causes almost 8,000 deaths each year) cell growth in a study in Nutrition and Cancer.

How to Use in Juicing

Juice your own tomatoes for a refreshing, healthy and tangy juice treat! Add garlic to tomato juice, it is a fantastic combination.

Flavor Enhancers for Juice

- ✓ Lemons and limes are great additions to your juice blends as they add fresh and tangy flavor and enhance the flavor of green vegetables, especially for those who do not find them palatable.
- ✓ Hot peppers can be juiced if you like spicy flavor.
- ✓ Fresh mint is a wonderful flavor for most any juice blend.
- ✓ You can stir in any spice you like once your juice is ready.
- ✓ Many herbs, like basil, and oregano can be juiced to get flavor and their respective health benefits.
- ✓ Add ice to make a cooler and refreshing drink.

- ✓ Some juicers allow you to make frozen drinks, a great idea for summer.
- ✓ Look up recipes online or in books to add variety to your juicing habit.
- ✓ Experiment with different fruits and vegetables to find you favorite blends. This is key is sticking with this healthy new habit!

Watch The Sugar Intake

Approximately 88% or more of all your juice blends should be vegetables, and 20% or less fruit.

Generally, best juicing practices prescribe the use of more vegetables than fruits as fruit is high in sugar.

Since it takes much more of the fruit to juice as it would if you were eating fruit whole, those who get into the habit of juicing more fruit than vegetables can easily triple or quadruple the recommended daily sugar intake for adults, not to mention calories with just one glass of juice.

Juicing When You Already Have Cancer

As part of your cancer fighting juicing diet, you should not eat any poultry, fish, meat, or dairy products. Cooked foods such as these prevent the immune system from maximally fighting off cancer cells. Instead, the immune system must spend its time dealing with the effects of cooked foods, pesticides, chemical supplements, fungicides, herbicides, toxins, and the hormones found in meat and dairy products. This prevents the immune system from fighting off cancer cells. Of course, you should consult with your doctor before making any dietary changes.

Don't eat a lot of fruits or vegetables that contain a lot of sugar unless they are one of the cancer fighting fruits and vegetables listed above. Carrot juice, for example, has a lot of sugar in it that is easily taken up by cancer cells. Along with the sugar, the cancer cells take up the cancer fighting nutrients from the carrots and are killed by the nutrients.

Juicing can be beneficial as a way to combat cancer when you already have the disease. When you are being treated for cancer, things like digestive issues, chewing, and swallowing are already problems you may be dealing with.

By juicing fruits and vegetables, you do not have to chew your food and the food is easily digested. You shouldn't go on an exclusively juiced diet, however, because it can result in weight loss, which is already a problem in people who have cancer.

Besides juicing, you should be eating at least five servings of whole colorful fruits and vegetables daily. You can eat these fruits and vegetables whole or juice some of them if you are having problems with digestion or swallowing.

Ideally, though, you should be eating the first five servings of fruits and vegetables, only juicing those you eat beyond that.

Tips On Juicing in Support of Cancer Treatment

Here are a few tips to juicing when you have cancer.

- **Eat more vegetables than fruits.** Vegetables contain the most cancer fighting phytonutrients so you should focus on those. You can add fruits to sweeten the juice but it should not make up the whole of the juice.

- **Drink the amount that you would eat.** If you are eating carrots, for example, it takes about 4-6 large carrots to make up to 8 ounces of carrot juice. This is a lot of carrots and more than you would likely eat if they were eaten whole. Only juice a couple of whole carrots at a time.
- **Add protein and fat to your diet.** Along with your juice (or in it), you should have some protein and healthy fats. This could mean that you eat yogurt with your juice or that you eat a handful of seeds or nuts. Eggs are also a good source of protein.
- **Don't forget the cruciferous vegetables**
- Arugula
- Broccoli
- Bok Choy
- Brussels Sprouts
- Cabbage
- Kale
- Radishes
- Rutabaga
- Turnips
- Watercress
- Cauliflower
- Collard Greens

These can be juiced or eaten whole and contain many cancer fighting phytonutrients. Try eating at least 3 servings of cruciferous vegetables in your diet every day.

Juicing for Skin Health

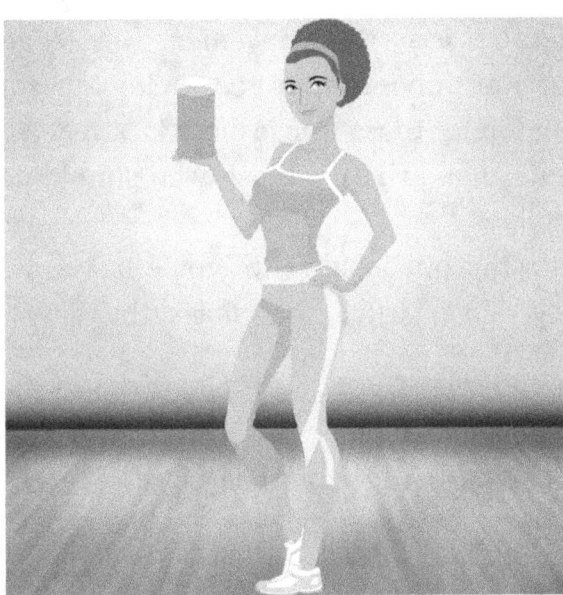

Good Skin Care

Healthy skin is beautiful skin and it all begins with good nutrition. Skin is an organ that requires nutrients just like every other part of our bodies to thrive, and remain healthy especially as we age.

That radiant healthy glow can be achieved with regular intake of plant foods that provide key vitamins, minerals and antioxidants that support the health of the skin.

Juicing for Healthy Skin

If you want healthy looking skin, look no further than juicing. There are many vegetables and fruits that can be juiced and are beneficial for your skin because they increase the amount of collagen in the skin. Collagen fills out the tissue beneath the skin so you have a reduced number of visible wrinkles.

Furthermore, fruits and vegetables are high in vitamins and minerals that fight the aging process that can be so unkind to the skin.

Of course, you should eat whole fruits and vegetables, but juicing offers an easy and convenient way to get a large infusion of nutrition into your body in liquid form. It is also a great option for those whose diet's lack vegetables and the nutrients they bring or those who simply don't like eating vegetables.

Juicing offers the opportunity to create tasty blends that include low sugar fruits that mask the flavor of vegetables.

Best Fruits and Vegetables for Healthy Skin

Cucumbers

Cucumbers are very high in water, in fact, they are mostly water, and they contain vitamin C, and caffeic acid that helps soothe irritations and swelling of the skin, which is why cucumbers are often recommended to be placed over swollen eyes to get rid of puffiness and a fatigued look when you have not had a restful night's sleep. Cucumber juice is very hydrating to improve skin moisture and being that vitamin C is one of the most important antioxidants, it can help your skin to maintain a youthful appearance.

Carrots

Carrots are extremely high in beta-carotene, which is a form of vitamin A. Beta carotene is perhaps one of the best antioxidants that prevents aging by reducing the degeneration of cells so you can maintain a youthful look. Vitamin A is also good for the growth of tissues, improved vision, healthy bones, and healthy teeth.

The vitamin C you'll find in carrots will increase the amount of collagen in the body and collagen improves skin's elasticity to prevent wrinkles and deflect the typical signs of aging.

Carrots are also high in potassium, which helps keep the electrolytes in the body balances, reduces acne, and increases the growth of healthy, new skin cells. Potassium can also relieve you of scarring as well as the dark spots so often seen in aged skin. Carrots help the liver get rid of toxins, which decreases the amount of acne you have on your skin.

Kale

Kale is one of the leafy green cruciferous vegetables that will help you fight acne. Kale is a food that Is considered anti-inflammatory and very healthy for you with loads of vitamins C, K, A, E, B1, B2, B3, beta carotene, calcium, iron, phosphorus, magnesium, copper, lutein (a carotenoid), omega 6 fatty acids and omega 3 fatty acids.

The vitamin A in kale will help repair and maintain the skin and the omega 3 fatty acids you find in kale will have anti-inflammatory properties. If you have skin conditions like acne, it may be because your colon isn't moving as

113

swiftly as it could. Juice up some kale to stimulate the bowels on a regular basis.

Beets

Beets are extremely healthy for your skin. They are high in nutrients that clean both the liver and the blood. You need clean blood in order to have clear skin. Because beets are an extremely potent vegetable, use just half a beet as part of the juice you make.

The micronutrients in beets that fight the aging properties of skin include potassium, iron, copper, vitamin C, niacin, magnesium, manganese, zinc, folic acid, and calcium.

Caution: You cannot eat beets or drink juices containing beets if you have kidney stones.

Parsley

Parsley is an herb that is high in vitamin A and vitamin C. Because of this, it helps maintain a normal skin tone and clears up acne blemishes. Besides its advantages for the skin, it cleanses the kidneys, liver, and urinary tract. You'll find high amounts of vitamin K in parsley, which improves the elasticity of the skin and increases the speed of wound healing.

Ginger

Ginger can be ground and juiced along with other healthy vegetables. It is a highly anti-inflammatory food that will help you fight acne blemishes. It also boosts your immune system so it fights off the bacteria that result in acne.

Ginger is high in anti-aging antioxidants as well as potassium, manganese, magnesium, and vitamin B6.

Watercress

Watercress will purify the blood, which makes it an excellent juicing choice for the skin. It is high in sulfur, which is a component that will improve your skin's complexion. Watercress is high in vitamin A, which is also good for your skin.

Watercress will help your liver work better and is high in anti-oxidants that fight the aging process in your skin. It will give you plenty of the daily requirements of vitamin K, vitamin C, B vitamins, beta-carotene, calcium, folate, and iodine.

Lemons

Lemons belong to the citrus family, so they have lots of vitamin C, B vitamins, and citric acid. It purifies the blood, which in turn clears up your skin. It also helps the body rid itself of toxins as well as cleans the kidneys.

Lemons are a great choice for juice as they are very low in sugar and add a lot of tangy flavor to vegetable juice blends.

Other Citrus Fruits

Besides lemons, you can brighten your skin with oranges, grapefruits, and limes.

They are high in vitamin C that helps the amino acids proline and lysine turn into collagen. You need the vitamin C as well to fight off oxygen free radicals, which can damage both collagen and elastin, increasing the wrinkling of the skin.

Tomatoes and Red Peppers

These red vegetables are high in the antioxidant called lycopene. Lycopene will help reduce the signs of aging of the skin by acting as a natural sunblock to protect the skin from the effects of UV radiation. It also increases the levels of collagen in the skin, reducing the appearance of wrinkles.

Spinach

Along with other dark, green vegetables, spinach is loaded with the anti-oxidant vitamin C, which can increase collagen levels. The anti-oxidant properties of spinach will fight against oxygen free radicals that helps prevent collagen from weakening.

Spinach juices great, and has so many other health benefits that it really is a great choice in juicing.

Berries

Berries like blueberries, raspberries, and black berries help scavenge for oxygen free radicals that can weaken collagen and can cause wrinkling of the skin. Berries are also high in free radical fighting antioxidants that are provide numerous anti-aging benefits for the body.

Garlic

You can spice up your juice with garlic, which is very high in sulfur. You need sulfur in order to make collagen in the body. Garlic is also high in taurine and lipoic acid, which are molecules that decrease collagen damage and increases collagen fibers.

Cabbage

You can make use of just about any kind of cabbage in a juicer, including bok choy, choy sum, cannonball cabbage, early jersey cabbage, Portugal cabbage, red drumhead cabbage, Napa cabbage, and savoy cabbage.

Cabbage contains many phytonutrients and antioxidants such as thiocyanates, lutein, isothiocyanates, zeaxanthin, and sulforaphane. These will hydrate the skin and will increase its elasticity.

Green Beans

Green beans are very healthy for your skin. They contain hyaluronic acid, which fights aging of the skin and hold onto water so the skin is moisturized thereby reducing wrinkles and fine lines. The skin is kept smooth and moist by the addition of hyaluronic acid.

Beans also increase the synthesis of collagen and promote the growth of healthy skin. Your joints are healthier and your skin will be more toned. Hyaluronic acid is also important in the proliferation of healthy skin cells and in the migration of those cells to the outermost parts of the skin.

Flaxseeds

Flaxseeds are high in omega 3 fatty acids that are healthful for the skin. You can substitute flaxseeds for walnuts to make your juice a little bit more substantial in texture. Walnuts are also high in omega 3 fatty acids.

Omega 3 fatty acids result in an increase in collagen production so you won't wrinkle as much and they also help decrease the chances that you will get skin cancer.

For juicing, stir in 1 or 2 teaspoons of finely ground flaxseed to any juice blend drink and enjoy the benefits!

Green or Black Olives

These can be juiced along with other fruits and vegetable. They are rich in sulfur, which helps increase collagen production. Sulfur has been used historically for a variety of skin conditions. It reduces the oiliness of skin so that pores aren't blocked and acne does not form from the blocked pores.

Avocado Oil

Avocados are added to smoothies, as they are rich in omega 3 fatty acids. Avocados are also high in plant steroids that are known to decrease the appearance of old age spots. Avocado oil is high in vitamin E, which is an antioxidant that protects the skin from suffering the damaging effects of oxygen free radicals.

You need omega 3 fatty acids to increase the production of collagen so that you can have beautiful skin. Because avocado oil is oily, it is good for people who have damaged dry skin because it regenerates and rejuvenates skin cells that have been damaged by the elements. Add 1 teaspoon to your juice blend for good skin health.

Hemp Seeds

Hemp seeds help improve the radiance and firmness of skin and they are the only edible source of linoleic acid (GLA) that provides omega-6 fatty acids that are part of the membrane around skin cells.

This protein rich plant food helps synthesize collagen and elastin to improve skin firmness and keep it looking supple. Ground hemp seeds can be easily added to juices and smoothies.

Prunes

Prunes are high in antioxidants that scavenge for oxygen free radicals that can result in premature aging of the skin. Prunes can be juiced along with other fruits or vegetables for some sweetness in the juice.

Plant Nutrition A to Z

Nutritional values and health benefits of all Fruits and vegetables.

Fruits

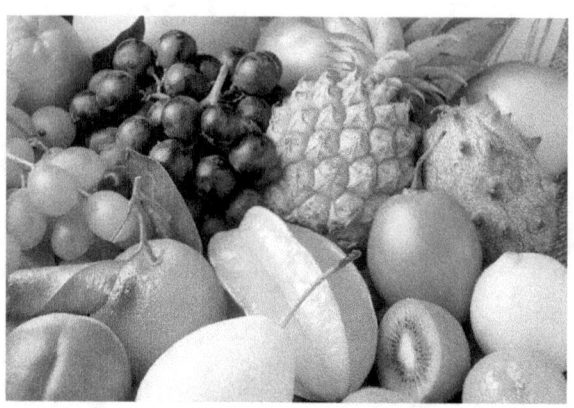

Apples

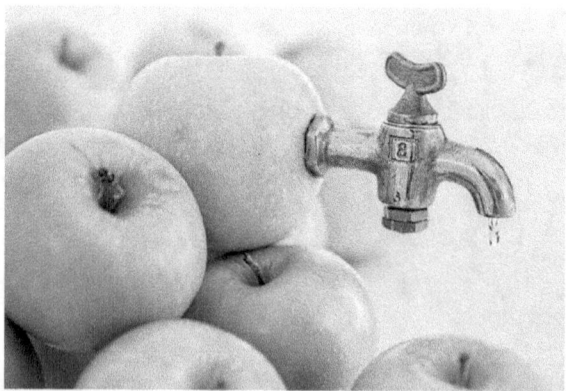

Key Nutrients
- ✓ Fiber (both soluble and insoluble types)
- ✓ Vitamins A, C, and E
- ✓ Potassium

Health Benefits

- May Reduce Development of Certain Types of Cancer- as if their delicious taste wasn't enough reason for you to start chomping down on apples, studies from the American Association of Cancer Research have demonstrated that their high flavone content contributed to reduction of pancreatic cancer cases by 23%. They also showed promise against colorectal cancer and breast cancer; but make note that the active constituents were all found in the peel.

- Decreases Likelihood of Developing Type 2 Diabetes- the high fiber content of apples likely contribute to thus, as it was shown that women were more than 28% less likely to develop diabetes over the course of their life given they eat an apple daily.

- Reduces Atherosclerotic Plaque- this is the residue that lines the blood vessel walls and plays a critical role in development of heart problems later in life. Apples also help control cholesterol levels, thanks to its fiber content and other phenolic derivatives found in the peel.

Apricots

Nutrients

✓ Vitamin C and A (particularly pro-vitamins called carotenoids)

✓ Minerals Potassium and Copper

✓ Fiber

Health Benefits

- Decrease Incidence of Age Relates Decline in Vision- although inevitable to an extent, the high content of carotenoids (Vitamin A like molecules) and other bio-flavonoids found in apricots, significantly slow down macular degeneration, help strengthen the optic nerve and preserve vision for much longer that it would left unmanaged.

- Boosts Skin Health- the phytonutrients found in apricots, along with its rich bioflavonoid levels promote synthesis of collagen in the body. In case you've never heard, as we age, collagen levels decrease, resulting in connective tissue (skin, cartilage etc.) weakening and drooping. That's why collagen supplements are so highly touted in skin health, as it preserves the suppleness of skin.

- Maintains Fluid Balance- apricots also contain high levels of potassium, a key, yet underrated mineral that keeps electrolyte levels in check. Without sufficient potassium, sodium levels go out of whack, resulting in dehydration, cramps, or even heart rhythm anomalies.

Asian Pears

Key Nutrients
- ✓ Vitamins C and K
- ✓ Copper
- ✓ Fiber

Health Benefits
- Deceased Risk of Certain Cancers- more specifically, colon-rectal cancer. The high content of soluble fiber in Asian pears is capable of binding with bile acids. High levels of bile acids have been shown to be associated with a higher risk of developing such cancers.
- Decreases Risk of Heart Disease and Developing Diabetes- once again, thanks to the high fiber content in Asian pears (both soluble and insoluble types) cholesterol forming bile acids can be neutralized, reducing production of such that can promote blockage of blood vessels. Asian pears are also rich in flavones, compounds with potent anti-oxidant and anti-inflammatory effects, that ravage free radicals before they can do damage to our bodies. Its fiber content keeps blood sugar levels stable, and insulin levels modulated, reducing diabetes risk.

Avocados

Key Nutrients
- ✓ Vitamins B5, B6, Folic Acid, Vitamin C, E and K
- ✓ Potassium

✓ Loaded with Good Monounsaturated Fats

Health Benefits

- Reduces Total Cholesterol and Triglyceride levels- a small study demonstrated that regular consumption of avocados reduced LDL (bad) cholesterol and triglyceride levels by 20%, while simultaneously increasing good HDL cholesterol more than 10%; very beneficial to heart health.

- May Promote Weight Loss- persons who consume avocados regularly report increased weight loss thanks to the hunger suppressing effect of fat, as well as its ability to promote fat burning.

- Boost Food Absorption- certain foods, especially plant based ones, are better absorbed in the presence of fat, thus making avocado an excellent vector to facilitate healthy absorption. You can eat the best food in the world, but if it is not getting absorbed by the intestines, it will be worth nothing.

Bananas

Key Nutrients
✓ Vitamin B6, C and Biotin
✓ Potassium, Copper, manganese
✓ Fiber

Health Benefits
- Helps Maintain Blood Pressure and Heart Function- thanks to its potassium content, sodium and water balance is kept in check ensuring no significant fluctuations to blood pressure.

- Reduces Cholesterol Levels- in addition to the cookie-cutter fiber content, bananas contain sterols, plant based cholesterol like compounds that have been shown to reduce cholesterol levels in humans.
- Can Help Maintain Physical Performance- athletes regularly consume bananas as a pre-workout meal, since it is a unique mix of water, electrolytes, carbohydrates and other vitamins that help to ensure energy levels remain stable throughout the activity.

Bitter Melon (Bitter Gourd)

Key Nutrients
✓ B Vitamins, Vitamin A and C
✓ Minerals Potassium, Zinc and Iron

Health Benefits
- Very Effective in Reducing Blood Sugar Levels and Useful in Diabetes- contains two plant compounds; polypeptide- P, which is a plant based insulin like compound, and charantin a compound that promotes glucose use and storage as glycogen not fat.
- Aids Digestion- useful in treating constipation and indigestion.
- May Decrease Cancer Risk- antioxidants contained in bitter melons may help scavenge free radical implicated in cancer development.

Black Currants

Key Nutrients
✓ Vitamins C, B and E
✓ Minerals iron, Phosphorus and Manganese

Health Benefits
- Reduce Likelihood of Alzheimer's Disease-polyphenols contained in black currants may play a role slowing down or preventing development of the debilitating disease altogether
- Kills Pathogens- studies conducted on infections of the upper respiratory tract displayed the potential of black currant extract in treating both bacterial and viral causes of such infections. The infective agent was unable to multiply, allowing the immune system the chance to handle the infection.
- May Reduce Symptoms of Arthritis- the anti-inflammatory potential of black currants may provide benefit to persons suffering from the joint disease who cannot use painkillers and other prescription anti-inflammatory medications.

Blackberries

Key Nutrients
✓ Vitamins A, C, E and K
✓ Minerals Copper, Iron and Magnesium
✓ Phyto-Nutrients Lutein and Zeaxanthin
Benefits for Health:

- Massive Anti-Oxidant Content- contains one of the highest antioxidants contents in the world, which is useful in particularly decreasing cancer risk.
- Helps Treat Inflammatory Bowel Conditions- including hemorrhoids, inflammation in the intestines and frequent diarrhea. This is due to the high tannin content of blackberries.
- Reduces Pain Associated with The Menstrual Cycle- blackberries have been consumed as a treatment for menstrual pain, which is thought to be as a result of the high Vitamin K levels in the fruit.

Blueberries

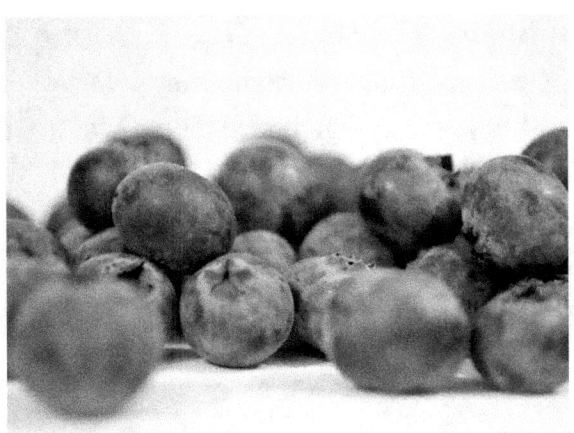

Key Nutrients
- ✓ Vitamins C and K
- ✓ Manganese
- ✓ Fiber

Benefits for Health

- Bone Health- contains many minerals and vitamins important in maintaining bone strength and integrity.
- Decreases Cancer Risk- known as one of the most anti-oxidant rich berries in nature, blueberries have found a place in preventing cancer development.

Boysenberries

Key Nutrients
- ✓ Vitamins A, B, C, E and Folic acid
- ✓ Minerals iron, potassium, manganese, calcium and phosphorus
- ✓ Protein

Benefits for Health
- Decreases Risk of Alzheimer's Disease- contains anthocyanins, which are beneficial in preventing age related brain degradation.
- Anti-Inflammatory- can reduce/relieve inflammatory conditions such as arthritis, or even plaque accumulation in blood vessels.

Cantaloupe

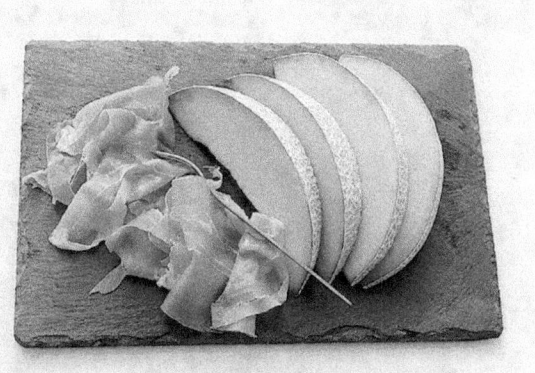

Key Nutrients
✓ Vitamins A, C and to a lesser extent B vitamins
✓ Potassium and Magnesium

Benefits for Health
- Hair and Skin Health- the high concentration of Vitamin A, along with Vitamin C, promotes healthy collagen production and keeps skin hydrated.
- Helps Keep Blood Pressure in a Normal Range- thanks to potassium, blood pressure is maintained within a normal range and so is sodium water balance.

Cherries

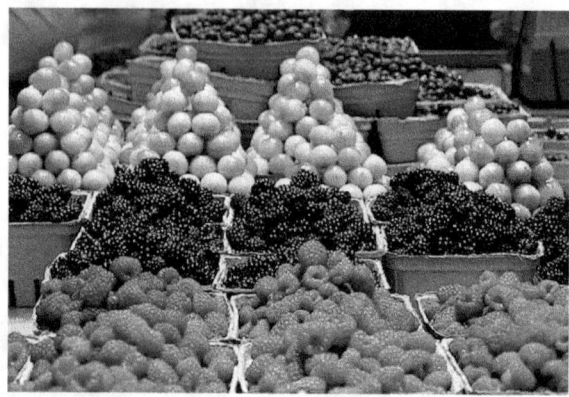

Key Nutrients
- ✓ Beta-Carotene (vitamin A pro-vitamin), Vitamin C
- ✓ Copper and Potassium
- ✓ Fiber

Benefits for Health
- Reduces Inflammation- can relieve pain as a result of swollen tissue, including arthritis or muscle damage.
- Boosts Eye Sight- contains lutein and zeaxanthin, two antioxidants important in maintaining optic function into adulthood.

Clementines

Key Nutrients
- ✓ Folic Acid and Vitamin C
- ✓ Minerals: Potassium, decent source of Magnesium and Calcium

Benefits for Health
- Boosts Brain Health- study conducted revealed that foods which contain a high concentration of folic

acid a folate promote brain function and can decrease the likelihood of depression occurring.

- Promotes Strong Bones and Muscles- minerals calcium, magnesium and phosphorus; all found in Clementines are important for bone health and normal muscular contraction. Even more important in the elderly.

Coconuts

Key Nutrients
✓ Minerals Manganese and Copper
✓ Extremely Key Nutrients saturated fatty acid Lauric acid
✓ B Vitamins

Benefits for Health
- Heart Health: promotes increase in beneficial HDL levels, reduces atherosclerotic plaque deposits in blood vessels, and decreases stroke risk.
- Excellent Hydrating Drink- coconut water is a good source of electrolytes, which was once used as saline in the Vietnam War. In addition, the water contains compounds known as Cytokinins, which have showed significant promise as anti-cancer therapies.

Grapefruits

Key Nutrients
✓ Vitamins A and C
✓ Potassium
✓ Lycopene

✓ Fiber

Benefits for Health

- Circulation and Heart Health- the combination of nutrients found in the grapefruit can help reduce triglyceride levels, helps maintain healthy blood pressure, and in a study was associated with a 49% lower chance of an ischemic event (stroke) occurring in women.

- Reduces Frequency of Asthmatic Attacks- citrus fruits contain high level of natural bioflavonoids, which reduce the frequency, or severity of asthmatic episodes.

Grapes/Purple Grapes

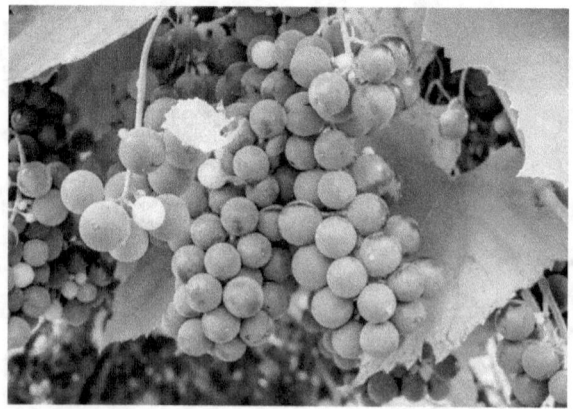

Key Nutrients
✓ Vitamins A, C and K
✓ Copper

✓ Resveratrol

Benefits for Health

- Anti-Aging and Cancer Prevention- the high concentration of antioxidants found in grapes, most importantly resveratrol, have shown immense promise in slowing the rate of telomere splitting, effectively slowing down aging. The reduced replication frequency of cells also translates to a diminished cancer risk.

- Diabetic Health- in addition to being low glycemic index, what is more interesting is its effects on diabetic nerve health. The nerve related degradation of the eye and peripheral limbs is reduced or reversed completely, likely by promoting blood flow to the nerves and preventing damage.

- Allergies and Asthma- bioflavonoids found in grapes are effective in reducing histamine response that triggers allergies and asthma, and can reduce severity of flare-ups when they do occur.

- Heart Health- grapes contain a compound called quercetin, which is an anti-inflammatory agent that reduces the rate of plaque formation in arteries. Phenol content in grapes can also help lower cholesterol levels and prevent platelet clotting.

Guavas

Key Nutrients
✓ Fiber

- ✓ Vitamins A, C and B9
- ✓ Minerals: Magnesium, Manganese, Potassium and Phosphorus

Benefits for Health
- Maintains Regularity- is effective in keeping bowel movements regular, and is used as a natural remedy for constipation as it adds bulk, but similarly is helpful in treating mild diarrhea for the same reason.
- Helps Prevent Certain Types of Cancers- loaded with antioxidants like all fruits, but also included lycopene, which adds another layer of protection. Is reportedly helpful in avoiding prostate and colon cancer.

Kiwifruit

Key Nutrients
- ✓ Vitamins C and E
- ✓ Folate
- ✓ Minerals: Potassium, Magnesium and Zinc
- ✓ Fiber

Benefits for Health
- Better Skin- contains Vitamin E, which is renowned for its effects on skin, as well as Vitamin C, which is an important precursor in collagen synthesis. Zinc also functions as an anti-oxidant to slow down aging.

- Improved Sleep- according to anecdotal evidence, the magnesium content in kiwifruit may help hasten onset of sleep and duration afterwards.

Lemons

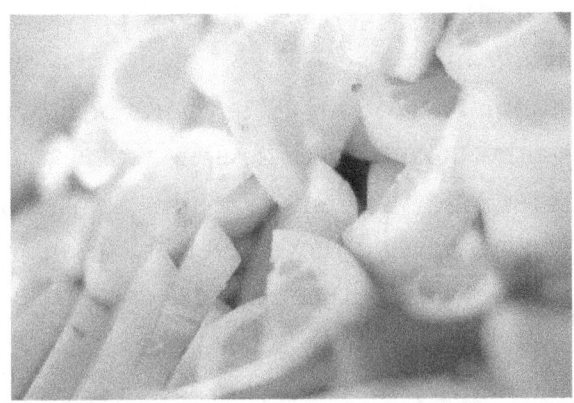

Key Nutrients
- ✓ Vitamin C and B6
- ✓ Potassium
- ✓ Fiber
- ✓ Bioflavonoids

Benefits for Health
- Heart Health- many botanical compounds found in lemons can help preserve cardiovascular function. For example, the compounds Hesperidin and Diosmin are antioxidants, which can strengthen blood vessel integrity, reduce inflammatory processes, and boost circulation.
- Arthritis – One study suggested that vitamin C-rich foods, such as lemons help to protect against inflammatory polyarthritis, which is a type of rheumatoid arthritis that affects two or more joints.

- Preventing Anemia- although most people first associate anemia treatment with an iron-rich diet, lemons do supply small amounts of iron. However, what makes it effective in addressing anemia is the presence of Vitamin C, which enhances the absorption of the little iron it possesses significantly.
- Immunity – vitamin C supports healthy immunity to prevent common illness, like colds and flu.
- Anti-septic - lemons also have anti-septic properties, and have been in used in natural healing for hundreds of years.

Limes

Key Nutrients
✓ Vitamin C
✓ Folate

Benefits for Health
- Reduces Risk of Cancer Development- while high Vitamin C intake is associated with a reduced risk of cancer, Limes are able to exert another anti-carcinogenic effect. Specific flavone glycosides, including many kaempferol-related molecules found in limes can modify or stop multiplication of cancer cells altogether. This effect is also beneficial in treating infections when the pathogen needs to multiply in number.
- Respiratory Disease- citrus bioflavonoids from many fruits have shown benefit in helping reduce allergen sensitivity.

Lychee

Key Nutrients
- ✓ Vitamin **C**
- ✓ Minerals: Potassium and Copper

Benefits for Health
- Red Blood Cell Formation- although Iron is the most well-known element involved in blood building, the Copper content of Lychees is also helpful.
- Keeps Skin Healthy- the benefits on skin can be attributed to two actions of the Vitamin C found in lychee; boost in collagen production, and the neutralization of harmful free radical, which bring about premature aging.

Mangos

Key Nutrients
- ✓ Vitamins A, C and B6
- ✓ Minerals: Copper, Potassium and Magnesium
- ✓ Fiber

Benefits for Health
- Alkalizes Blood pH- acidic blood pH has been implicated in many inflammatory conditions, including cancer and heart disease. The body's natural pH is closer to basic, so mangos are a great addition to normalize levels.
- Helps with Memory and Concentration- mangos have high levels of glutamic acid, an amino acid important for healthy brain function.

Nectarines

Key Nutrients
- ✓ Vitamins A, B, C and E
- ✓ Minerals: Potassium, Calcium, Magnesium and Phosphorus

Benefits for Health
- May Help with Weight Loss- nectarines contain two efficient weight loss agents, catechins, and chlorogenic acid derivatives. These compounds boost metabolism and lipolysis.
- Eye Health- nectarines contain the important anti-oxidant lutein, which have shown importance in preserving optic nerve function, and preventing age related macular degeneration.

Oranges

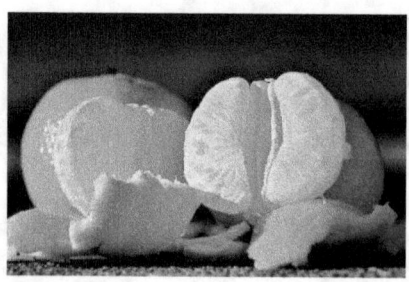

Key Nutrients
- ✓ Fiber
- ✓ Vitamins C and B
- ✓ Minerals: Copper, Potassium and Calcium

Benefits for Health
- May Help in Prevention of Kidney Stones- the citric acid content in oranges is able to help prevent the

development of kidney stones, by binding with excess calcium levels in blood before they are filtered by the kidneys.

- Reduced Risk of Certain Cancers- the Vitamin C content coupled with other active botanicals in oranges have demonstrated potential in reducing the risk of cancers, especially of the colon.

Papayas

Key Nutrients
✓ Vitamins A, and C
✓ Folate
✓ Fiber
✓ Minerals: Magnesium, Potassium and Copper

Benefits for Health

- Promotes Healthy Digestion- in addition to being Key Nutrients dietary fiber, which is important for maintaining regularity, papaya contains a much sought after digestive enzyme, papain, which aids in the digestion and subsequent absorption of food, especially protein based.

- Prevents Premature Aging- loaded with a bevy of antioxidants, collagen boosting agents, as well as essential Vitamins, regular consumption of papaya can have marked benefits on skin.

Passion Fruit

Key Nutrients
- ✓ Vitamins A, C, Niacin and Riboflavin
- ✓ Minerals: Potassium, Iron, Magnesium and Copper
- ✓ Fiber

Benefits for Health
- Improves Blood Circulation- minerals potassium and copper and known for having mild vasodilatory effects; when coupled with iron that boosts blood production, the result is enhanced circulation.
- Respiratory Disease- the purple colored variety of passion fruit peel had demonstrated expectorant and bronchodilatory (relaxing) effects on respiratory organs. This can be especially helpful in people suffering from asthma, COPD, or chronic bronchitis.

Peaches

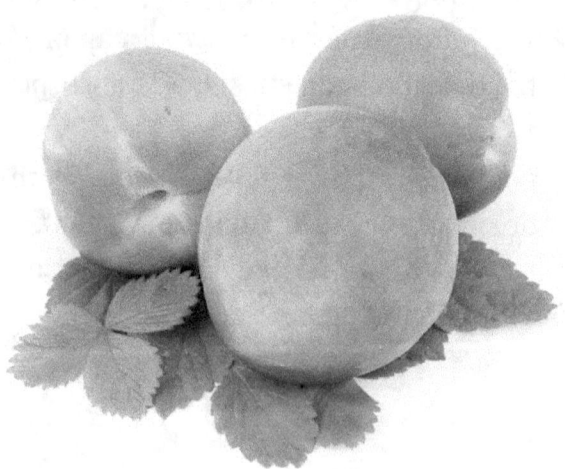

Key Nutrients

- ✓ Vitamins A and C
- ✓ Minerals: Potassium, Iron and Magnesium
- ✓ Fiber

Benefits for Health

- Eye Health- presence of antioxidants helps prevent macular degeneration and weakening of the optic nerve, helping preserve vision for a longer time.

- May Have Utility in Cancer Treatment- it is well established by now that fruits of all types have the tendency to reduce cancer risk, but in addition to this, a study revealed that extracts from peaches and plums killed out aggressive breast cancer cells, heralding what could possibly be a big breakthrough in cancer treatment.

Pears

Key Nutrients
- ✓ Fiber
- ✓ Copper
- ✓ Vitamin C and K

Benefits for Health

- Digestive Support- the fiber content in pears is easily digestible, and is one of the reasons pear is stomach friendly. However, pears are easily digested, and are recommended by doctors for patients after recovering from surgery for this same reason. They are even considered "hypoallergenic" fruits because of the very low incidence of allergies or adverse effects from eating them.

- Helps Support Blood Sugar Levels- pears are low glycemic fruits, meaning that they do not cause a rapid conversion to sugar and subsequent insulin spikes. In addition, the presence of multiple flavonoids and fiber further helps to slow down and sustain the release pattern of the sugar in the fruit, and other foods taken around this time.

Persimmons

Key Nutrients
✓ Fiber
✓ Vitamins A, B6, C and E
✓ Potassium

Benefits for Health
- Boosts Eye Health- Persimmons are an excellent source of several antioxidants important for eye health, including lutein, zeaxanthin, and lycopene. In addition to preventing age related decline, they can also help prevent the development of cataracts.
- May Reduce Cholesterol Levels- a study conducted revealed that the use of persimmon extract, standardized for tannins led to a reduction in blood cholesterol levels. This can decrease your cardiac risk of heart disease.

Pineapple

Key Nutrients
✓ Vitamins B and C
✓ Minerals: Manganese and Copper

✓ Fiber

Benefits for Health

- Co-Enzyme Production- pineapple supplies several important trace minerals, which are important in the synthesis of enzymes and immune bodies. Lack of sufficient mineral intake could lead to a compromised immune system with varied symptoms ranging from the lungs to the colon.

- Digestive Support- pineapple supplies a decent amount of fiber, but also the much sought after enzyme Bromelain. Similar to Papain (the enzyme found in Papayas), Bromelain helps with digestion, most important of which is protein. Persons consuming a high protein diet find bromelain to be very important in achieving nutritional goals.

Plums

Key Nutrients

✓ Vitamins A, B. C, E and K
✓ Minerals: Calcium, Magnesium, Zinc, Potassium, Phosphorus, Iron and Fluoride
✓ Fiber

Benefits for Health

- Prevents Obesity Related Disorders- plums play a role in reducing inflammatory conditions within the body, but especially in obese patients. Metabolic syndrome does not develop as readily, and can slow down the development of diabetes, high blood pressure, or elevated cholesterol levels.

- Reduces Anxiety- the chlorogenic acid content in plums can play a role in exerting anxio-lytic effects, or by preventing oxidation to pathways that trigger anxiety attacks.

Pomegranates

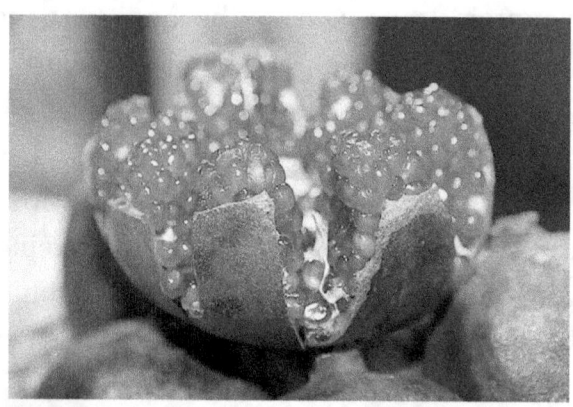

Key Nutrients
- ✓ Fiber
- ✓ Vitamins C, K and Folate
- ✓ Potassium

Benefits for Health
- Extremely Potent Anti-Inflammatory Effect- this is thanks to the presence of two unique compounds, Punicalagins and Punicic Acid. These compounds can significantly reduce the likelihood of cancer, Diabetes, heart conditions; Alzheimer's or even Obesity from developing.
- Relieve Symptoms of Arthritis – While other anti-inflammatory foods help this condition, the pomegranate provides the added benefit of blocking the production of enzymes that contribute

to degenerative joint conditions, allowing regeneration, and recovery. Trials are currently preliminary, but this fruit remains a hopeful alternative to common treatments used today.

Raspberries

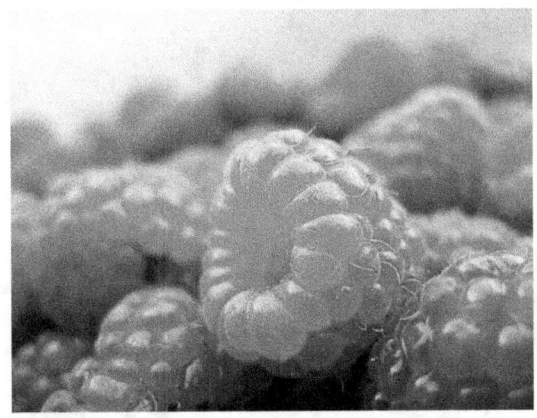

Key Nutrients
- ✓ Vitamins B, C, K and E
- ✓ Minerals: Copper, Manganese, Potassium and Magnesium
- ✓ Omega -3 Fatty Acids
- ✓ Fiber

Benefits for Health
- Obesity Prevention/ Reduction- studies conducted demonstrate the potential of compounds in raspberries (better known as raspberry ketones) to have actions relating to increasing metabolism in fat cells or decreasing their absorption by the body. Thus, it can both prevent subsequent obesity as well as reduce body fat levels above optimal levels.

- Cancer Prevention- raspberries have been consumed for years in the effort to prevent cancer development. Additionally, it was revealed that berries farmed organically possess superior anti-oxidant effects by virtue of their concentration of flavonoid and Anthocyanidins compounds.

Red Currants

Key Nutrients
✓ Fiber
✓ Vitamin B6, C and K
✓ Minerals: Iron, Magnesium and Calcium

Benefits for Health
- Boosts Red Blood Cell Production- anemia is extremely common, yet undiagnosed in the majority of patients. It can be simply avoided by consumption of iron rich foods, in addition to supporting c-nutrients needed for production of blood. Red currants provide a basic amount of these nutrients, and can help to maintain already normal levels.
- Keeps Skin Healthy- red currants contain antioxidants, which help neutralize harmful free radicals, vitamins to aid in collage synthesis, and can help neutralize the damaging effect of UV radiation on the skin.

Strawberries

Key Nutrients
✓ Fiber
✓ Vitamins C, B6, Folate
✓ Minerals: Iodine, Potassium, Manganese and Copper
✓ Modest Omega-3 Fatty Acids

Benefits for Health
- Antioxidant and Anti-Inflammatory Effects- strawberries are ranked among the best anti-oxidant fruits in the world, possessing massive antioxidant concentration of Vitamins, phytonutrients and minerals that assist in the synthesis of the important anti-oxidant enzyme super oxide dismutase (SOD).
- Blood Sugar Reduction- interestingly, the effect of blood sugar modulation is not related to its fiber content, but rather the presence of an enzyme known as alpha-amylase. Our bodies contain amylase, which breaks down sugars into simple glucose for absorption. Strawberries prevent this breakdown, and subsequent absorption, restricting the degree and inulin spike can peak. Very helpful in preventing insulin resistance from developing.

Tangerines

Key Nutrients
✓ Vitamins A, C and Folate
✓ Potassium

✓ Fiber

Benefits for Health

- Restrict Absorption of Fat from Foods- the fibers in Tangerines have the ability to limit how much fat is absorbed from a meal. These fibers are known as pectin and hemi-cellulose.
- May Speed Up the Healing Process- the antioxidants contained in tangerines, as well as folate, which is responsible for normal DNA and RNA replication, ensures wounds heal properly and faster.

Tomatoes

Key Nutrients
✓ Vitamins A, B, C and E
✓ Minerals: Molybdenum, Potassium, Copper and Phosphorus
✓ Fiber
✓ Lycopene

Benefits for Health

- Supports Bone Health- a recent study remonstrated the importance of antioxidants on bone health; using the restriction of tomatoes (with lycopene) as the test. Researchers noticed increased rates of oxidative bone damage following weeks of restriction, leading to the conclusion that lycopene and ant-oxidants do play an important role in bone health, in addition to ensuring that enough nutrients are being supplied.

- Reduces/ Treats Prostate Cancer- though more research needs to be conducted before a definitive conclusion can be made, preliminary studies have demonstrated that a compound in tomatoes known as alpha-tomatine, has been used successfully to reprogram cancer cells of the prostate, to commit "suicide" a process known as apoptosis. The compound can also profoundly alter the metabolic processes of these cancerous cells.

Best Eaten Raw When You Need Vitamin C – Cooking can destroy vitamin C in both fruits and vegetables, including tomatoes. Testing conducted by Rui Hai Liu, an associate professor of food science at Cornell University found that vitamin C declined 10% when tomatoes were cooked for 2 minutes and 29% when they were cooked for 30 minutes at 190.4 degrees.

The reasons this occurs is vitamin C is highly unstable, and easily degraded when exposed to heat, oxidation, and through cooking in water. However, since tomatoes contain lycopene, which is more difficult to find in other produce, and which is boosted by the cooking process, it may be a worthwhile trade off, especially since you can get your vitamin C from various sources, including, carrots, citrus fruits, cauliflower, broccoli and kale.

Watermelon

Key Nutrients
✓ Vitamins A, B and C
✓ Minerals: Potassium, Copper and Magnesium
✓ Citrulline

✓ Lycopene

Benefits for Health

- Improved Blood Flow- one of the most important compounds in watermelon, known as L-citrulline, converts to an important vasodilatory agent in the body, better known as L-Arginine. L-arginine enhances blood flow around the body, and is effectively used as an adjuvant to treat men suffering from erectile dysfunction.

- Antioxidant Effect- watermelon contains a battery of unique phytonutrient anti-oxidant, one of the most interesting being Cucurbitacin E. This agent is able to inhibit action of the enzyme COX, which is responsible for synthesis of prostaglandins, and unique free radicals called reactive nitrogen species (RNS).

Vegetables

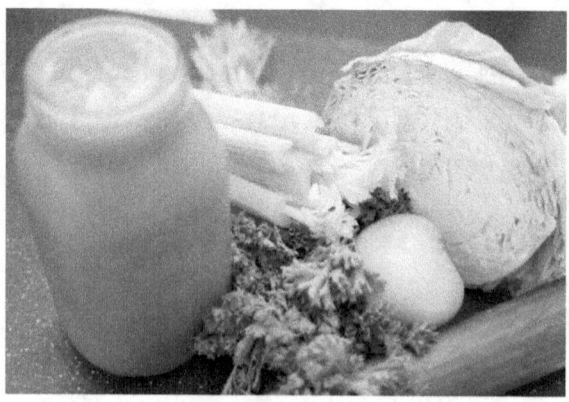

Artichokes

Key Nutrients
✓ Vitamins A, B, C, D, E and K
✓ Minerals: Calcium, Zinc, Magnesium and Potassium
✓ Fiber

Benefits for Health
- Liver Detox and Recovery- artichokes are related to milk thistle, an herb classically used to treat disorders of the liver. Artichokes contain silymarin, which speeds up removal of toxins from the body, helps aid liver recovery, and returns to normal elevated levels of liver enzymes.
- Cancer Prevention- according to a study conducted by the USDA, artichokes have the highest anti-oxidant content of any vegetable, and rank 7 overall in terms of density of these compounds. As such, regular consumption can play a large role in helping diminish the chance of cancer development.

Asparagus

Key Nutrients
✓ Vitamins K, B, C, E and A
✓ Minerals: Copper, Selenium and Manganese
✓ Fiber

Benefits for Health
- Unique Digestive Support- when most people think of digestion support they are envisioning

the stomach, or the small intestine to a lesser extent. However, what makes asparagus particularly interesting is the presence of a special carbohydrate known as inulin, better known as a prebiotic. This carb is not digested in the stomach of small intestine, but rather in the large intestine, where it acts as a food source for the probiotic bacteria acidophilus and lactobacillus. These bacteria are associated with improved digestion, decreased risk of food allergies, and even a reduced chance of colon cancer.

• Anti-Inflammatory and Antioxidant Effects- asparagus contains an immense number of anti-oxidant compounds, some not found in any other plant on earth. Of particular interest is one compound known as sarsasapogenin, which shows promise in treating ALS (Lou Gehrig's disease), which is believed to have a significant inflammatory process. In addition, asparagus contains significant levels of the powerful anti-oxidant glutathione, which is important for keeping oxidation levels on cells low, as well as providing liver support for efficient detoxification.

Beets

Key Nutrients

✓ Vitamin C and Folate
✓ Fiber
✓ Minerals: Manganese, Potassium and Copper

Benefits for Health

- Longevity- beets contain many dual anti-oxidant and anti-inflammatory compounds, which exert numerous Benefits for Health. However, studies have determined that the benefits gained from beets are individual, since only about 15% of persons in the US are regarded as "responders" (able to gain maximum benefits of these compounds).

- Supports Detox- removal of toxic metabolite from cells is essential, as accumulation of these waste materials could pave the way for a battery of diseases and disorders. Beets have been shown to stimulate the action of a key detox compound, glutathione, which bonds to the waste molecules and facilitates easy excretion of urine or stool.

Pro Tip: Many of the compounds found in Beets are not stable in the presence of heat; as such, it is important to make note of cooking times. If steaming, expose to heat for a maximum of 15 minutes, and roasting, 1 hour. Any longer and you risk losing the bulk of nutritional benefits.

Bell Peppers

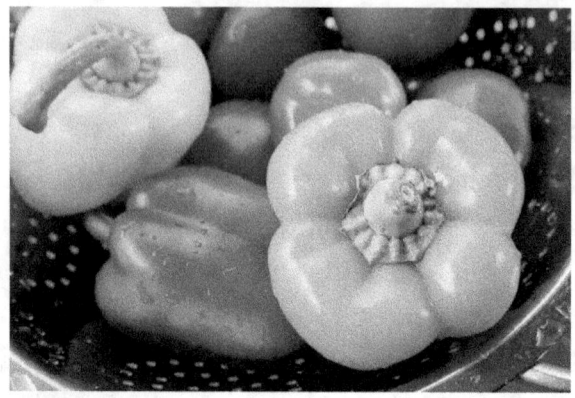

Key Nutrients
- ✓ Vitamins A, B, C, E and K
- ✓ Minerals: Molybdenum, Potassium, manganese
- ✓ Fiber

Benefits for Health
- Anti-Cancer Benefits- though not confirmed by multiple studies, there was research conducted on compounds found in bell peppers referred to as cysteine S-conjugate beta-lyases. These compounds are important in Sulphur metabolism, which is another important detox pathway that is implicated in the genesis of cancer.
- Antioxidant benefits- loaded with a ton of antioxidant nutrients, regular consumption of bell peppers can help preserve vision, and diminish the risk of cardiovascular disease or diabetes.

Best Eaten Raw: Bell peppers quickly lose concentrations of antioxidant compounds when exposed to heat. When grilled for just 7 minutes under high heat, there was an overall reduction of levels by more than 40%.

Red bell peppers also contain about 150% of the daily-recommended value of vitamin C, but the National Institutes of Health warns that this vital nutrient breaks down when the peppers are cooked at or above 375 degrees Fahrenheit. Eating raw red peppers also helps prevent atherosclerosis that leads to heart disease.

Black Eyed Peas

Key Nutrients
✓ Potassium, Zinc and Iron
✓ Fiber
✓ Modest protein levels for vegetarians

Benefits for Health
- Modulate Blood Sugar Levels- black eyed peas contain high amounts of soluble fiber, which helps to keep blood sugar levels stable, and prevent massive insulin spikes.
- Boost Heart Health and Blood Pressure- Key Nutrients potassium, which keeps heart muscles healthy, maintains normal sodium-water balance, and acts as a vasodilator to blood vessels keeping pressure normal. Iron content also contributes to blood cell production, which improves circulation and supply of oxygen rich blood.

Black Radishes

Key Nutrients
- ✓ Vitamins A, B, C and E
- ✓ Potassium, Iron and Magnesium

Benefits for Health
- Maintains Thyroid Function- studies of one of the active constituents found in Black Radishes, known as Raphnin have revealed that it can help modulate both over and under efficiency of the thyroid gland, helping keep metabolism in its optimal range.
- Boosts Resistance to The Common Cold- black radishes are popular during winter months, primarily because of their immune boosting properties. Loaded with anti-oxidant vitamins, along with its potential to up the defense of mucous membranes and relieve congestion.

Bok Choy
(Also Known as Pak-Choi or Bak Choi)

Key Nutrients
- ✓ Vitamins K, C and A
- ✓ Minerals: Potassium, Calcium, Manganese and Iron
- ✓ Fiber
- ✓ Omega-3 Fatty Acids

Benefits for Health

- Keeps Bones Healthy- you may be surprised to know that Bok Choy does more for your bones than milk ever could, thanks to the presence of Vitamin K and antioxidants, which research has shown can have a protective effect on bones.
- Boosts Immunity- in addition to the presence of the many antioxidants found in most vegetables, the presence of the trace mineral selenium in Bok Choy aids in the production of specialized Killer T cells, which are incredibly efficient at removing foreign invaders from the body.

Broccoli/Broccolini

Key Nutrients
- ✓ Vitamins A, B, C and E
- ✓ Chromium, Phosphorus, Manganese, Potassium and Copper
- ✓ Fiber
- ✓ Omega-3 Fatty Acids
- ✓ Protein

Benefits for Health
- Heart Defense- Broccoli supports a healthy heart via some unique mechanisms not possessed by other vegetables; it does so in 3 key ways.
- Broccoli Promotes Excretion of Bile Acids and Lowers Cholesterol- bile acids need to be produced from cholesterol, but is typically recycled, negating the need to use more cholesterol. Broccoli promotes its excretion, prompting the body to

make more bile from cholesterol, thus reducing the overall stores of cholesterol in the body and thus levels.

- Maintains Blood Vessel Integrity- most people do not understand how blockages occur. In short, whenever the body notices a minor blood vessel tear or damage, platelets and other compounds aggregate there, forming a "plaster." Over time, more and more residue starts to accumulate there, leading to a significant reduction in the diameter of the vessel at that area. That is the start of heart disease. A compound in broccoli called glucoraphanin is able to prevent or reverse the damage to these vessels, preventing the necessity of an aggregation response to such alarming extents.

- Lowers Levels of Key Heart Disease Risk Factor Homocysteine- the B vitamins broccoli provides is able to remove excessive levels of homocysteine found in our body, reducing the risk of stroke, heart attack, and atherosclerotic plaque thickening.

- Detoxification – few foods are capable of providing comprehensive detoxification in our bodies, since this usually involves 3 phases. Broccoli compounds are able to enhance detoxification on the cellular level, making the process far more efficient that merely injecting more antioxidants at a random stage.

Best Eaten Raw or Lightly Steamed: Eating raw broccoli helps fight cancer. Chewing raw broccoli allows you to access a cancer-fighting compound known as myrosinase, which is easily killed off in the cooking process. Eating broccoli sprouts doubles your intake of anticancer properties.

Like tomatoes, broccoli contains high levels of vitamin C that is destroyed when it is cooked for 29 minutes or more, according to testing conducted by Rui Hai Liu, an associate professor of food science at Cornell University.

Brussels Sprouts

Key Nutrients
- ✓ Vitamins A, B, C and K
- ✓ Minerals: Manganese, Copper, Potassium and Iron
- ✓ Fiber
- ✓ Omega-3 Fatty Acids
- ✓ Protein

Benefits for Health
- Digestive Support- the high fiber content, along with the many potent antioxidants, decrease the risk of digestive issues arising or indigestion occurring.
- Detox- Brussels sprouts contain many antioxidants can offer support comparable to broccoli. In addition, the presence of omega-3 fatty acids helps to balance the levels of pro-inflammatory Omega-6.

Pro Tip: Similar to Broccoli, some phytonutrients in Brussels sprouts become more efficient after heating. For example, it's cholesterol reducing components become approximately 33% more efficient at removing bile acids after being cooked (preferably steamed).

Cabbage

Key Nutrients
- ✓ Vitamin B, C and K
- ✓ Fiber
- ✓ Minerals: Manganese, Potassium and Copper

Benefits for Health

- Cancer Prevention- thanks to cabbage's rich anti-oxidant and anti-inflammatory content, which would normally be enough to significantly reduce the risk of cancer. However, in addition, cabbage contains compounds known as glucosinolates, which have proved cancer preventative for many different types of cancer.

- Cholesterol Reduction- by increasing excretion of bile acids, and prompting new production from cholesterol, blood cholesterol levels are reduced.

Pro Tip: If you want to take full advantage of cabbage's cholesterol lowering effect, consume it steamed. Steam helps to activate more of the bile-acid binding components, so that greater excretion ensues.

Cactus

Key Nutrients
- ✓ Minerals: Calcium, Magnesium and Manganese
- ✓ Fiber
- ✓ Vitamins A and C

Benefits for Health

- Promotes Healthy Digestion- the high fiber content of cactus as well as its high natural water content

160

promotes regularity and can ease digestive disturbance.

- Helps Control Diabetes- in addition to its high fiber content that blunts blood sugar spikes, it may inhibit the liver from releasing excessive sugar into the blood stream at any one time. This is helpful when dieting to lose weight or improve insulin sensitivity.

Carrots

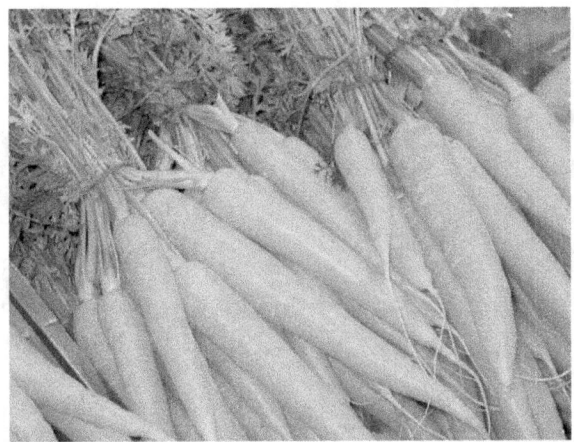

Key Nutrients
- ✓ Vitamins A, B, C and K
- ✓ Minerals: Molybdenum, Potassium, Manganese
- ✓ Fiber

Benefits for Health
- Eye Health- the benefits of Vitamin A antioxidant compounds on eye health has been proven, as persons who frequently consume carrots have lower incidence of glaucoma, along with macular degeneration.

- Heart Health- carrots contain many anti-inflammatory phytonutrients that are useful in preventing abnormal aggregation of platelets in blood vessels, especially in the coronary arteries.

Cauliflower

Key Nutrients
- ✓ Vitamins B, C and K
- ✓ Fiber
- ✓ Omega-3 Fatty Acids
- ✓ Manganese and Phosphorus

Benefits for Health
- Detox Support - cauliflower, like broccoli and Brussels sprouts, possesses significant detox properties of both phase 1 and phase 2 processes.
- Reduces Cancer Risk - antioxidants and other phytonutrients found in cauliflower reduce the likelihood of cancer via multiple mechanisms.

Celery

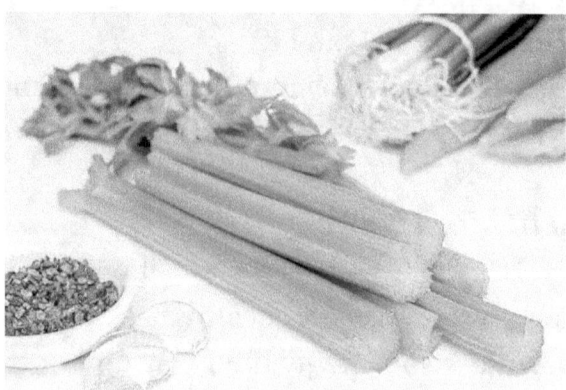

Key Nutrients

- ✓ Vitamins B and K
- ✓ Molybdenum, Potassium and Manganese
- ✓ Fiber

Benefits for Health

- Digestive Health- some of the compounds found in celery actively protects the stomach from inflammation or development of peptic ulcers.
- Heart Health- celery boasts numerous anti-inflammatory compounds, which help to preserve blood vessel wall integrity, and can lead to a state of vasodilation or blood vessel relaxation.

Chives

Key Nutrients
- ✓ Vitamins A, C and K

Benefits for Health

- Decreases Cholesterol Production- compounds found in chives have been found to possess activity similar to prescription medication that inhibits an enzyme in the liver that synthesizes cholesterol.
- Reduces Likelihood of Alzheimer's Occurring- Vitamin K has been associated with decreasing the risk of developing Alzheimer's disease.

Cilantro

Key Nutrients
✓ Vitamin A and K

Benefits for Health
- Powerful anti-inflammatory capacities that may help symptoms of arthritis
- Protective agents against bacterial infection from Salmonella in food products
- Acts to increase HDL cholesterol (the good kind), and reduces LDL cholesterol (the bad kind)
- Relief for stomach gas, prevention of flatulence and an overall digestive aid
- Wards off urinary tract infections
- Helps reduce feelings of nausea
- Eases hormonal mood swings associated with menstruation
- Has been shown to reduce menstrual cramping.
- Adds fiber to the digestive tract
- A source of iron, magnesium, and is helpful in fighting anemia
- Gives relief for diarrhea, especially if caused by microbial or fungal infections
- Helps promote healthy liver function.
- Reduces minor swelling
- Strong general antioxidant properties
- Disinfects and helps detoxify the body
- Stimulates the endocrine glands
- Helps with insulin secretion and lowers blood sugar

- Acts as a natural anti-septic and anti-fungal agent for skin disorders like fungal infections and eczema
- Contains immune-boosting properties
- Acts as an expectorant
- Helps ease conjunctivitis, as well as eye-aging, macular degeneration, and other stressors on the eyes.

Collard Greens

Key Nutrients
- ✓ Vitamins A, B, C, E and K
- ✓ Minerals: Manganese, Iron, Copper and Calcium
- ✓ Fiber
- ✓ Protein

Benefits for Health
- Lowers Cholesterol Levels- collard greens possess the highest cholesterol lowering effect of any cruciferous vegetable, being able to promote the excretion of bile acids most efficiently.
- Reduces Cancer Risk- via presence of powerful phytonutrients, collard greens assist the detox and anti-inflammatory pathways in the body to eliminate toxins, keep oxidation manageable and limit the potential of cells to turn cancerous.

Corn

Key Nutrients
- ✓ Vitamin B

✓ Fiber
✓ Phosphorus and Manganese

Benefits for Health

- Promotes Healthy Growth of Intestinal Flora- corn is composed of both insoluble and soluble fiber, which bacteria in the large intestine use as nourishment. This promotes healthy growth of cells in this area, reducing cancer likelihood.
- Controls Blood Sugar Levels- once again, by virtue of its fiber levels, corn is able to buffer blood sugar spikes and allow for a more uniformed absorption process.

Cucumbers

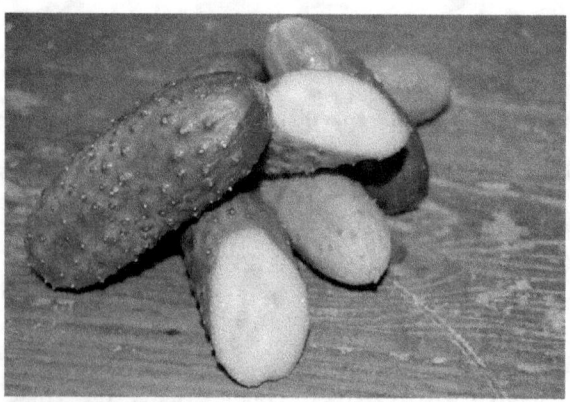

Key Nutrients
✓ Vitamins K and B
✓ Moderate Levels of Vitamin C
✓ Molybdenum and Potassium

Benefits for Health

- Anti-Cancer Potential- compounds known as lignans found in cucumber and cruciferous vegetables have shown excellent promise in preventing cancers in the lab, especially breast and prostate cancers.
- Stomach Health- compounds found in the cucumber are able to inhibit a pro-inflammatory enzyme known as COX-2.

Eggplant

Key Nutrients
✓ Fiber
✓ Copper and Manganese
✓ Vitamin B

Benefits for Health
- Brain Health- the skin of eggplant was found to contain a compound called nasunin, which is able to cell membranes in the brain from oxidation and damage.
- High Chlorogenic Acid Levels- this is a phenolic compound that provides anti-cancer, anti-viral and cholesterol lowering effects.

Endive

Key Nutrients
✓ Vitamins A, B, C and K
✓ Fiber
✓ Calcium, Potassium, Manganese and Zinc

Benefits for Health

- Promotes Healthy DNA Synthesis- endives have a high concentration of folates, which are essential to maintain normal DNA replication patterns.
- Anti-Cancer Potential- endives contain compounds called kaempferol, which have been shown to inhibit the growth of cancer cells themselves, as well as restricting the growth of new blood vessels, a mechanism cancer cells use to continue growing.

Fennel

Key Nutrients
- ✓ Vitamin C
- ✓ Molybdenum, Potassium and Manganese
- ✓ Fiber

Benefits for Health

- Cancer Prevention- fennel contains numerous anti-oxidant compounds, most notable of which is one called anethole. Anethole is capable of shutting down cancer signaling pathways, making cells insensitive to stronger carcinogenesis triggers.
- Controls High Blood Pressure- compounds in fennel, including potassium, can reduce the influence of sodium on water retention, allow blood vessel relaxation, and consequently decrease blood pressure.

Garlic

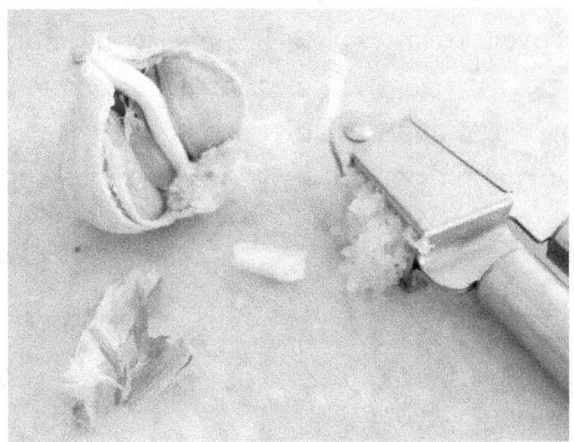

Key Nutrients
✓ Manganese, Copper and Selenium
✓ Vitamin B6 and C

Benefits for Health
- Relieves Arthritic Pain- compounds found in garlic can relieve inflammation caused by arthritic joints.
- Reduce Obesity- garlic shows promise in inhibiting a stage in obesity genesis not well known. Immature fat cells need to mature before their fat retention potential is amplified, a scenario believed favored by inflammatory conditions. Garlic can inhibit this maturation along with the inflammatory stage that needs to be set.

Best Eaten Raw: Freshly raw chopped garlic contains the enzyme alliinase that converts alliin into allicin, which is what creates the specific aroma of fresh garlic and also helps to improve your health. According to the University of Maryland Medical Center, allicin has antifungal, antibacterial, and antiviral properties.

Moreover, fresh raw garlic releases a short-lived gas known as hydrogen sulfide that acts as an intracellular signaling compound that protects the heart. Cooking, processing, and drying destroy this valuable compound.

Green Beans

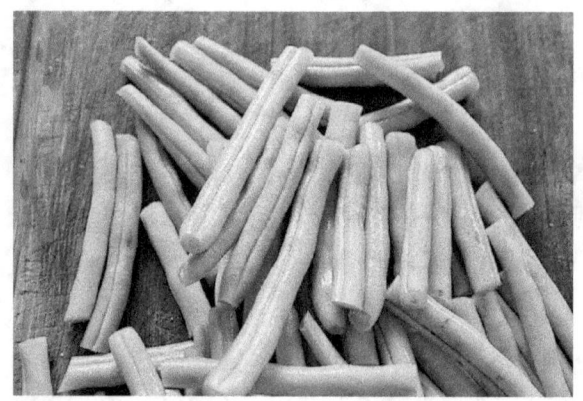

Key Nutrients
- ✓ Vitamins B, C and K
- ✓ Minerals: Manganese, Copper and Magnesium
- ✓ Fiber

Benefits for Health
- Decreases Inflammatory Processes- inhibits the action of several pro-inflammatory enzymes, including COX and lipo-oxygenase.
- Eye Health- green beans contain a high proportion of carotenoid compounds, which are essential to eye health.

Pro Tip: To retain maximum nutritive value, it is recommended to cook via steaming for a maximum of 5 minutes. This also reportedly brings out their flavor the best.

Kale

Key Nutrients
- ✓ Vitamins A, B, C, E and K
- ✓ Minerals: Manganese, Copper and Calcium
- ✓ Fiber

Benefits for Health
- Comprehensive Detoxification- kale is able to modify body detox on a genetic level, improving efficiency significantly.
- Cancer Reduction- kale's cancer preventative ability has now been proven in 5 different types of cancer including prostate, bladder, colon, breast and ovarian.

Kohlrabi
Key Nutrients
- ✓ Fiber
- ✓ Vitamins A, C, B and K
- ✓ Minerals: Copper, Magnesium and Potassium
Benefits for Health
- Neuro-Muscular Health- thanks to its high potassium content, Kohlrabi ensures that electrical signals are conveyed properly from nerve to muscle to elicit movement. Also helps to prevent cramping.
- Preserves Vision- the high beta-carotene content in kohlrabi helps to prevent or slow down age related

breakdown, glaucoma, or even cataracts in some cases.

Leeks

Key Nutrients
- ✓ Vitamin K and Folate
- ✓ Manganese and Copper

Benefits for Health
- Cardiovascular Health- one of the compounds in leeks, kaempferol, can help minimize or heal vascular injury, preventing the need for many aggregants to adhere to a damaged section of the vessel. This aggregation significantly promotes the development of atherosclerotic plaques.
- Arthritis- leeks show promise in treating osteoarthritis and rheumatoid arthritis, which have inflammatory components beneath their development.

Lettuce (all types)

Key Nutrients
- ✓ Vitamins B, A and K
- ✓ Molybdenum ,Potassium and Manganese

Benefits for Health
- Prevents Deposit of Plaque On Artery Walls- when cholesterol is oxidized, it contributes significantly to the process of atherosclerosis occurring. Lettuce contains potent antioxidants, which prevent

oxidation of cholesterol. In addition, the fiber content in lettuce is able to promote excretion of bile acids, prompting the usage of cholesterol to make more bile.

- Prevents Constipation- in addition to its high fiber content which keeps regularity in check, lettuce also has a high water volume, coming in handy for people who struggle with getting enough water in their diet.

Mushrooms

Key Nutrients
✓ Copper, Selenium and Zinc
✓ Vitamin B
✓ Fiber
✓ Modest amounts of Vitamin D

Benefits for Health
- Cardiovascular Support- mushrooms contain compounds that are uniquely able to target molecules, which promote adhesion on blood vessel walls, such as in the case when micro tears occur and platelets and a host of immune factors converge. By inhibiting the release of this "sticky" molecule, the majority of aggregants will be unable to converge at the spot, making the scab much smaller than would otherwise occur.
- Immune Support- mushrooms are interesting in the way they support the immune system, simply because they can either stimulate or diminish its

abilities. For example, mushrooms may stimulate the action of macrophages, which are important for identifying foreign bodies, including cancer cells. On the other hand, they may reduce immune expression in cases like rheumatoid arthritis, when the body actively produces antibodies against its own joints.

Okra

Key Nutrients
✓ Fiber
✓ Vitamins A, C, K and Folate
✓ Iron, Manganese, Magnesium and Calcium

Benefits for Health
- Lowers Cholesterol- its high levels of fiber, containing a rare mucus bases polysaccharide makes okra very effective in lowering cholesterol levels.
- Controls Diabetes- diabetics with poorly controlled blood sugar levels can benefit from regular consumption of okra since it retards the speed of absorption of sugar into the blood stream.

Onions

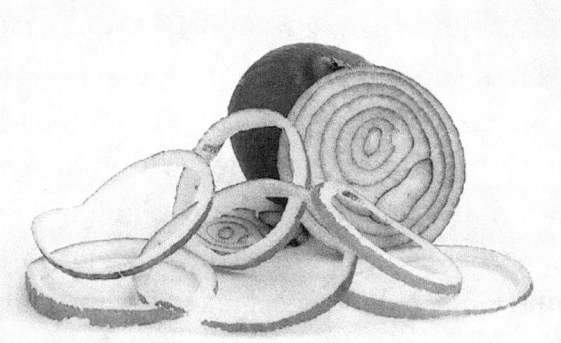

Key Nutrients
- ✓ Vitamins B and C
- ✓ Manganese and Copper
- ✓ Fiber

Benefits for Health
- Bone and Joint Health- the high Sulphur content of onions, coupled with their nutrient profile and anti-oxidant potential can help prevent age associated bone loss, or joint degradation. Since Sulphur is an important part of the connective tissue of joints, onions may also possess advantages for cartilage regeneration as well.
- Cancer Prevention- onion has been shown to decrease the risk of various cancers even when consumed in moderate quantities weekly. It is believed that higher levels of consumption also translate to added layers of protection from various cancers.

Pro Tip: Precise peeling of the outermost layer of the onion contributes to maximum retention of the nutrients contained within. Peeling too thickly can result in loss of over 75% of some beneficial compounds found closely underneath the outer peel.

Best Eaten Raw: A Cornell University study found that raw onions contain sulphur compounds, and cancer-fighting antioxidants that are only present in their juice. These nutrients help protect against lung and prostate cancer.

Parsnips

Key Nutrients
- ✓ Vitamins C and Folate
- ✓ Manganese, Potassium and Magnesium
- ✓ Fiber

Benefits for Health
- Healthy Growth- consumption of folates is important in growing children as deficiency could impair the necessary replication of cells needed to promote growth.
- Healthy Metabolism- in addition to folate, parsnips contain small amounts of other V vitamins, which help optimize metabolism of foods, and consequently increase your energy levels.

Potatoes

Key Nutrients
- ✓ Vitamins B and C

- ✓ Minerals: Manganese, Potassium, Phosphorus and Copper
- ✓ Fiber

Benefits for Health
- Healthy Metabolism- potatoes contain high levels of vitamin B6, which play important roles in various enzymatic processes integral to energy production.
- Reduces Blood Pressure- contain compounds called kukoamines which have the potential for assisting with blood pressure reduction in patients in conjunction with prescription medication.

Pumpkin

Key Nutrients
- ✓ Vitamins A, C and E
- ✓ Fiber
- ✓ Minerals: Potassium, Copper and Manganese

Benefits for Health
- Eye Health- one of the most established benefits of pumpkin consumption is on visual health. Its massive Vitamin A content helps preserve visual acuity and can offset the likelihood of acceleration degradation.
- Pumpkin Seeds Are Good Sources of Plant Based Omega-3 Fatty Acids- pumpkin seeds contain decent levels of omega -3 fatty acids that contribute

to synthesis of many anti-inflammatory compounds in the body, as well as helps prevent enlarged prostate conditions from occurring.

Radishes

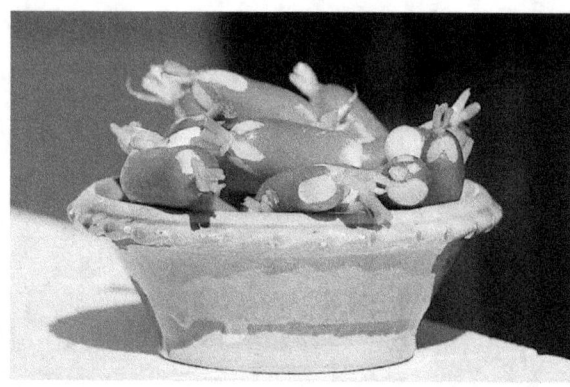

Key Nutrients
✓ Vitamins C and Folate
✓ Potassium and manganese

Benefits for Health
- Aids in Liver Detox- very helpful in treating jaundice or related conditions as it can help with removal of bilirubin for excretion. Also very effective in helping with cellular detox.
- Treats Urinary Disorders- radishes promote diuresis, reduce inflammation and burning during urination.

Rhubarb

Key Nutrients
✓ Vitamins K and C
✓ Potassium, Manganese and Calcium

✓ Fiber

Benefits for Health

- Promotes Bone Health- the nutrients in rhubarb can stimulate growth of new bone, as well as limiting breakdown of existing bone.
- Aids Intestinal Discomfort- including constipation, bloating or even cramping due its fiber content.
- One of the lowest sugar content fruits so ideal for juicing and a sweet tooth, especially when trying to lose weight.

Sprouts

- **Alfalfa Sprouts** - Vitamins A, B, C, and E, Calcium, Carotene, Magnesium, Potassium, Iron, Zinc, and Chlorophyll
- **Adzuki Sprouts** - Vitamins A, C, and E, Niacin, Iron, and Calcium
- **Buckwheat Sprouts** - Vitamins A, C, E, Calcium and Lecithin
- **Clover Sprouts** - Vitamins A, B, C, and E, Calcium, Zinc, Magnesium, Potassium, Iron, and Trace Elements
- **Fenugreek Sprouts** - Vitamin A, Iron, Niacin, Calcium
- **Garbanzo Sprouts** - Vitamins A, C, and E, Calcium, Iron and Magnesium

- **Lentil Sprouts** - Vitamins A, B, C, and E, Calcium, Iron and Phosphorus
- **Mung Bean Sprouts** - Vitamins A, C, and E, Iron and Potassium
- **Pea Sprouts** - Vitamins A, B, and C
- **Radish Sprouts** - Vitamin C, Chlorophyll and Potassium
- **Sunflower Greens** - B Complex Vitamins, E, Phosphorus, Potassium, Magnesium, Calcium, Iron, and Chlorophyll
- **Wheat and Rye Sprouts** - B Complex Vitamins, Vitamins C, and E, Phosphorus, Magnesium, and Pantothenic Acid
- **All Sprouts Are Great Sources of Protein**

Benefits for Health

Sprouts are nature's prefect food, because they are still in their early growth stage, they provide high levels of nutrients, key enzymes and vitamins, all ready to be digested by the human body.

Best Eaten Raw

Spinach

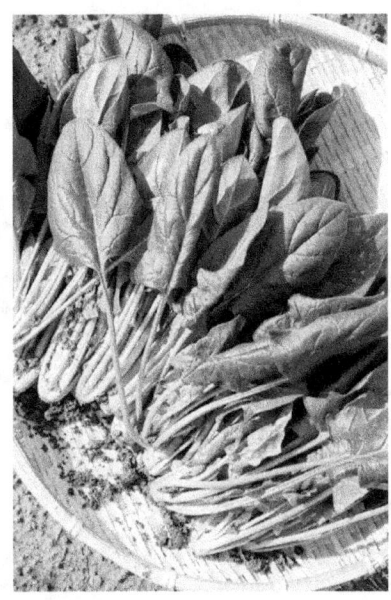

Key Nutrients
✓ Vitamins A, B, C, E and K
✓ Manganese
✓ Iron
✓ Copper
✓ Calcium
✓ Potassium
✓ Fiber

Benefits for Health
- Maintains Clear Blood Vessels- compounds found in spinach prevent oxidation of cholesterol, which subsequently forms plaque on the insides of blood vessel walls.
- Promotes Brain Health- research has found that compounds found in spinach can help retain brain

function over time, and delay or prevent the onset of Alzheimer's disease.

Squash

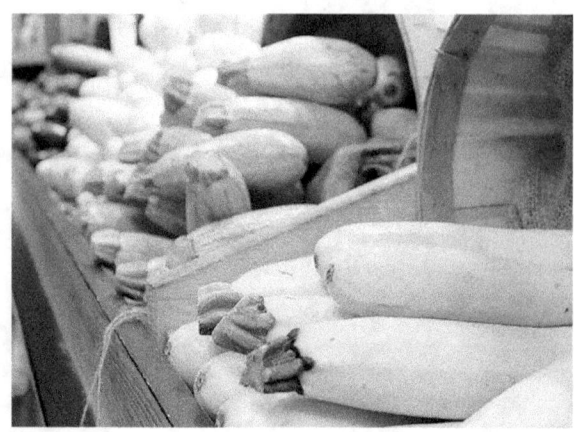

Key Nutrients
- ✓ Vitamin s A. B, C and E
- ✓ Magnesium, Potassium and Manganese
- ✓ Fiber

Benefits for Health
- Regulates Blood Sugar Levels - compound called d-chiro-inositol is believed responsible for control of blood sugar levels.
- Skin Health - squash is a water rich vegetable, which in conjunction with its vitamin and mineral content contributes to skin health.

Sugar Snap Peas

Key Nutrients
- ✓ Vitamins C, A, K and Folate

✓ Manganese and iron
✓ Fiber

Benefits for Health
- Reduces Cravings- can help modulate blood sugar levels with high fiber levels. Since they have a sweet flavor, they can reduce the desire to consume additional sweets.
- Boosts Regularity- their high fiber content contributes to regularity and prevents accumulation of waste in the colon.

Sweet Potatoes

Key Nutrients
✓ Vitamins A, B and C
✓ Minerals: Potassium, Manganese and Copper
✓ Fiber

Benefits for Health
- Reduced Cancer Risk- sweet potatoes are extremely Key Nutrients the potent anti-oxidant vitamin A, which contributes to prevention of cellular mutations.
- Helps Regulate Blood Sugar Levels- sweet potatoes have a low glycemic index, and are loaded with fiber which make it the perfect accompaniment to any meal, or better yet for a diabetic. In addition, if baked then consumed with the skin, further benefits have been observed for diabetics.

Swiss Chard

Key Nutrients
- ✓ Vitamins K, A and C
- ✓ Magnesium and Manganese

Benefits for Health
- Improved Athletic Performance- consumption of Swiss chard leaves have been associated with improved oxygenation levels of cells, allowing for more intense workout sessions.
- Improves Blood Pressure- Swiss chard contains key minerals that help to relax blood vessels, helping to maintain normal levels.

Turnips (Root and Leaves)

Key Nutrients - Root
Vitamin C
Key Nutrients – Turnip Leaves
- ✓ Vitamins K, A, B, E and C
- ✓ Copper, Manganese, Calcium
- ✓ Fiber

Benefits for Health
- Detoxification Support- turnip greens are particularly effective as detox support, not so much the roots. The leaves can provide support for the first two phases of detoxification.

- Digestive Health- provides enough fiber to ensure that regularity is maintained, and also possesses an important compound that helps regulate the population of H-Pylori bacteria residing in the stomach, overgrowth of which can lead to painful ulcers.

Watercress

Key Nutrients
✓ Vitamins K, C and A

Benefits for Health
- Cancer Prevention- compounds found in watercress leaves, called isothiocyanates, are show to blunt the action of carcinogens on normal cells.
- Bone Health- its vitamin K content supports bone health.

Zucchini

Key Nutrients
✓ Vitamins B and C
✓ Potassium and manganese
✓ Fiber

Benefits for Health
- Prevents Symptoms of BPH- BPH is a men's condition afflicting the prostate gland which results in overgrowth. Zucchini contains compounds,

which inhibit the conversion of testosterone to dihydrotestosterone, the hormone that "feeds" the enlarged cells.

- Heart Health- concentration of potassium and anti-oxidant vitamin C help to keep blood vessels dilated and free of oxidized cholesterol, which subsequently reduces the risk of a cardiac episode.

Recipes

Recipes for Exercise

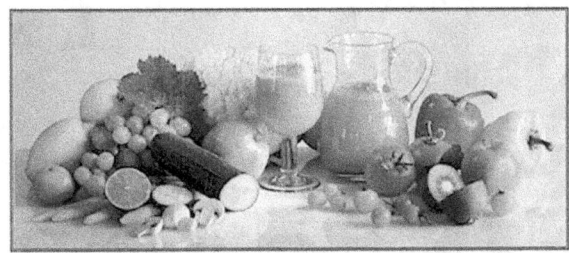

10 Workout Boosting Juicing Recipes

Here are some great juicing recipes to power your workouts. These recipes pack a lot of punch and they will fuel your pre and post-workout routines.

Preparation of these juices will depend on your juicer model, as they are all different in requirements for cutting, speed settings and order in which to juice.

Get juicing!

Magnesium Magic

Too many of us don't get enough magnesium, yet this micronutrient plays an essential role in a solid workout. If you're looking to find a way of sneaking more of this mineral into your diet, this represents a fantastic way to do so.

Ingredients:
- Large Handful of Parsley
- 3 leaves of chard
- 1 Cup Watermelon
- 4 carrots
- 1 Peach

- 2 Celery Stalks Including the Leafy Tops
- 1 Lemon

Dynamite Blend

Stop reaching for a sports drink after your exercise, and start making this antioxidant-and vitamin C rich juice instead. It's super rich in all your essential vitamins and minerals.

Ingredients:
- 1 Orange
- 2 Kale Leaves (or collard greens leaves)
- 1 Green Apple
- 1 Lemon
- 1 Lime
- 4 Broccoli Florets (including stems and leaves)

Repair and Recovery

This is nature's best antidote for aiding recovery so that you can go again soon. It helps to repair muscle and tissue damage and makes your body tougher over the long-term.

Ingredients:
- 1 Green Apple
- ½ Cup Strawberries
- ½ Pound of Organic Tart Cherries
- 2 Celery Stalks
- 4 Kale Leaves
- ½ Cucumber
- ½ Lemon

The Red Resurrector

Tomato juice is super rich in electrolytes, and ideal for maintaining proper hydration during and before a workout. Tomatoes also have many other health benefits and essential antioxidants to prevent chronic disease.

This juice includes an added boost from coconut water, which is naturally rich in electrolytes, so you can skip the sports drink and get your energy from juice instead.

Ingredients:
- 1 Lemon
- 5 Medium Carrots
- 2 Tomatoes
- 1 Cucumber (super hydration)
- Handful of Cilantro
- 1/ Cup of Coconut Water

Beet Power Juice

Ingredients:

- 3 carrots
- 3 kale leaves
- 1 Beet Including Leafy Tops
- 1" Piece of Fresh Ginger
- 1 Garlic Clove
- 1 Lime
- ½ Grapefruit

Post Workout Bliss Juice

Another great all natural post-workout recovery blend.

Ingredients:

- 2 Beets (nitric-oxide to oxygenate the blood)
- 2 Pears
- 1" piece of ginger (anti-inflammatory)
- 1 Handful of Spinach (strong bones)
- 1 cucumber (super hydration)

Pre-Workout Energy Blast Juice

Get all the energy you need for your intense workouts with this refreshing blend.

Ingredients:

- 3 Beets
- 2 Large Carrots
- 2 Green Apples
- 2" Piece of Fresh Ginger
- 1/4 Lemon
- 1/4 Lime

Iron Infusion Juice

This juice is loaded with healthy iron rich vegetables for healthy production of hemoglobin, healthy red blood cells, and fighting fatigue.

Ingredients:

- 1 Apple
- 1 Orange
- 6 to 7 Spinach leaves
- 1/2 Beet Including the Leafy Tops

Green Iron Power Juice

Another iron rich blend, with super healthy greens and ginger that fights inflammation.

Ingredients:

- 35 Spinach Leaves
- 25 Sprigs of Fresh Mint
- 15 Sprigs of Fresh Coriander
- 1/2 Lime
- 1" Piece of Ginger
- 1/2 Lemon

Vitamin D Infusion Juice

Get your vitamin D fix from this blend.

Ingredients:

- Handful of Kale leaves
- Handful of Spinach Leaves
- 1 kohlrabi
- 1 Cucumber
- 1 Mango
- 1 Grapefruit
- 1 Peach

Anti-Aging Juicing Recipes

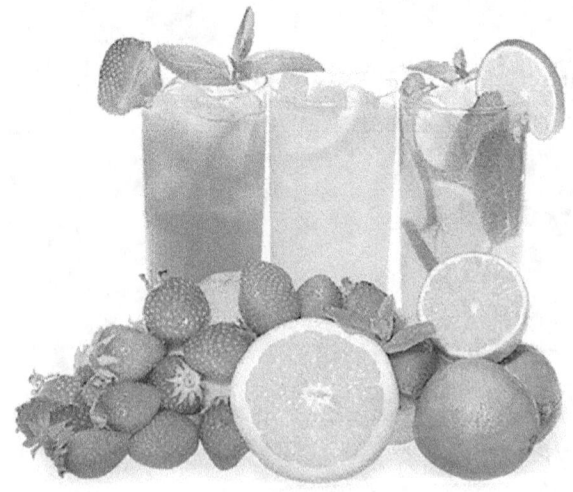

Sweet Greens

- 4 Kale Leaves

- 1 Green Apple
- 4 Celery Sticks
- 8 Parsley Sprigs
- 1 Cucumber
- ½ Peeled Lemon

Carrot Spice Juice

- 7 Carrots
- 1" Piece of Ginger (Peeled)
- ½ Lime
- ¼ Cup Cilantro
- Pinch of Cayenne Pepper (Add to Finished Juice)

Beet Treat

- 1 Carrot
- 1 Beet
- 1 Pineapple Ring That Is About One Inch Thick
- ½ Peeled Lemon
- 2 Granny Smith Apples
- 1 Piece of Ginger, Peeled and ½ Inch Thick

This makes for a healthy juice that is red in color because of the beets.

Antioxidant Boost Juice

This juice is loaded with vitamins A and C and provides you with more than the recommended daily allowance for vitamin K, which is good for bones and the blood.

- Handful of Kale
- Handful of Green Grapes
- 1 Cucumber
- 1 Green Apple

Anti-Aging Boost Juice

This juice provides powerful antioxidants that can fuel all the cells of your body and fight the aging process. Vitamin C, vitamin A, and lutein increase collagen production thereby reducing the signs of aging.

- 1 Apple
- 1 Bunch of Purple Grapes
- 1 Bunch of Collard Greens
- ½ Cup Pitted Cherries

Antioxidant Smoothie

Loaded with berries that have loads of antioxidants to fight off oxygen free radicals in your cells for better cellular health and it has only 151 calories. Blend the ingredients in a blender, food processor or any smoothie making machine, these ingredients are better blended than juiced.

Blend

- ½ Cup of Strawberries
- ½ Cup of Blueberries
- ½ Cup of Mango
- Use Water, almond milk, coconut milk/water, raw milk or a vegetable juice for liquid.

Muscle Juice

This juice will provide you with plenty of protein to feed and promote lean muscle mass that is key in healthy aging and weight management. Sweet potatoes provide lots of potassium, an essential mineral for cardiovascular health and turmeric has more than 100 health benefits.

- 1 Orange
- ½ Cup of Sweet Potatoes
- 2 Apples (any kind you like; the red varieties will be more sweet)
- 3" Piece of Fresh Turmeric
- 2 Stalks of Celery
- 3 Teaspoons of Finely Ground Almonds (stir in with a spoon after juice is done)

Energy Blast

- 3 Carrots
- 1 Small Green Apple
- 1 Peach
- 1/2 Lemon
- 1" Piece of Ginger
- 1 Handful of Mint Leaves

Lycopene Bliss

Tomatoes have high amounts of beta-carotene and lycopene that help reduce risk for cancer and heart disease. They taste magnificent when juiced fresh at home.

- 2 Large Tomatoes
- 1/2 Cucumber
- 1/2 Cup Cilantro
- 1/4 Lemon

Immunity Booster

Fresh ginger has many health benefits; it helps boost immunity, digestion, and blood circulation. Kale contains isothiocyanates, another immunity-boosting compound making these leafy superstars a go to for good health.

- 3 Carrots
- 1 Bunch of Kale
- 1" Piece of Ginger (peeled)
- 1 Small Green Apple

Wheatgrass Harmony

- 3 Stalks of Celery
- 2 Cucumbers
- 5 Spinach Leaves
- Cup Fresh Parsley
- 2 Ounces Fresh Wheatgrass Juice

Juice all ingredients except wheatgrass, dilute with water as needed. Add wheatgrass juice and blend.

Optional: Add ½ a lemon or 1 green apple for flavor to diminish the intensity of the vegetables.

Spinach Energy Blast

A refreshing and high-energy blend to get you going no matter your age.

- 5 To 6 Ounces Baby Spinach Leaves
- 2 Celery Sticks
- 1 Sprig of Mint
- 1/2 Large Lemon
- 1 Green Apple
- 2 Medium Carrots
- 2" Piece of Ginger

Beet Renewal

This juice is loaded with antioxidants and 1100mg of potassium, good for the body and anti-aging for the skin.

- 5 Celery Stalks
- 4 Beets Including the Leaves
- 2 Cups Red Grapes (Stems Removed)
- 3 Carrots

Watermelon Breeze

Watermelon is a great skin hydrator as it is 80% water and it contains high amounts of vitamin A and vitamin C, which boosts immunity.

Watermelon is also low in sugar and so this juice is ideal for a treat when losing weight.

- 2 Cups of Watermelon

- 1 Cup of Strawberries (can be juiced or blended and added to the final juice blend)
- 1/2 Fresh Lime
- 1" Piece of Fresh Ginger

Recipes for Healthy Skin

Carrot Ginger Juice

This is juice is high in beta-carotene from the carrots, but it also contains apples, which clear up the skin and add sweetness to the juice.

Ingredients:

- 4 carrots
- ½ apple
- 1" Piece of Ginger

Skin Brightening Juice

This is a juice that works for any skin type. It contains parsley, which detoxifies the system and stimulates the lymph system to reduce water retention. The spinach has omega fatty acids (alpha-linolenic acid and linoleic acid), that helps skin glow. Green apples are better for the skin than red apples and will both tone and brighten the skin. This makes for a dark green juice that is sure to protect your skin from damage and keep it bright and toned.

Ingredients:
- 4 Carrots
- Handful of Parsley
- ½ Green Apple
- Handful of Spinach

Pineapple Skin Brightening Juice

Pineapple is high in the enzyme bromelain, which is good for both the skin and for digestion. Bromelain is so good for the skin that it is often used as a topical agent in masks used to exfoliate and clear the skin.

The cucumber and apple in the juice will purify the skin and increase the alkalinity and hydration of the tissues. The combination of ingredients acts as an anti-inflammatory, which will decrease the inflammation you often see with acne. It can also be applied as a facial to the skin.

Ingredients:
- ½ Cup Fresh Pineapple

- 1 Cucumber
- ½ Green Apple

Dry Skin Relief Juice

This juice is high in vitamin C and antioxidants, which protect the skin from the effects of oxygen free radicals.

Ingredients:
- 1 Medium Green Apple
- 1 Small Cucumber
- 1 Beet
- 3 Medium Carrots
- 2 Oranges
- ½ Lemon

Optional: Stir in half a teaspoon of avocado oil to finished juice.

Homemade V8 Juice

This combination of vegetables will make your skin glow, and will free it of lines and wrinkles. It increases the collagen level of the skin and contains antioxidants, which fight oxygen free radicals intent on doing damage to the skin.

Ingredients:
- 2 Kale Leaves
- 1 Collard Green Leaf
- Handful of Fresh Parsley
- 1/2 Red Bell Pepper

- 1 Stalk of Celery
- 1 Carrot
- 1 Broccoli (Including Stems, Leaves and Floret)
- 1 Large Tomato

Optional: Juice 1 hot pepper with above ingredients or add 1 teaspoon of dried cayenne pepper spice.

Vitamin E Skin Nourishing Juice

This juice includes vitamin E rich vegetables that nourishes and moisturizes the skin.

Ingredients:

- 1 Green Apple
- Bunch of Spinach
- Bunch of Swiss Chard
- ½ Lemon

Optional: Stir in 1 teaspoon of very finely ground sunflower or sesame seeds to the finished juice to get more vitamin E.

Peach and Basil Juice for Dry Skin

This is an especially good juice for dry skin. It is high in vitamin C, which acts as an antioxidant to protect the skin from oxygen free radicals.

Juice the ingredients in this order:

1. 3 Leaves of Fresh Basil
2. ½ Lemon
3. 5 Medium Peaches
4. 7 Medium Carrots

Green Juice Recipes

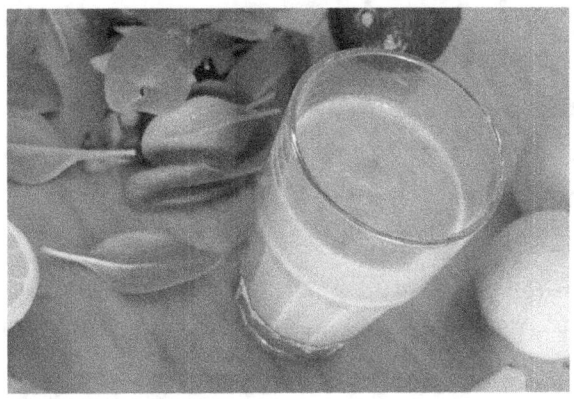

Green Energy Juice

It's easy to juice; simply push all the above ingredients into your juicer and go for it. It's incredibly energizing, and does more you're for health, wellbeing and mental alertness than your usual cup of coffee. It's a fantastic way to start the day.

Ingredients:

- 5 Kale Leaves
- 3 Cups Spinach
- 1 Green Apple
- 1" Piece of Ginger
- 1 Sprig of Mint

Sweet Berry Green Juice

Here is a very simple green recipe where the sweet antioxidant rich berries blend perfectly with the nutrient dense kale.

How to:

1. Juice 5 Kale leaves
2. Blend 1 cup of any berries you like, strawberries, raspberries, etc. You can use a blender, a food processor or just mash the berries with a fork if time allows.

Add the berry puree to your kale juice, mix with a spoon, and enjoy!

Optional: For added zing, and to boost the nutrient content, juice ½ a lemon or lime with the kale, and/or juice a 1" piece of ginger.

Oh My Sweet Basil

Ingredients:
- 1 Handful of Basil Leaves
- 1 Apple
- 1 Cucumber
- ¼ Lime
- 3 Spinach Leaves

Juice everything, starting with the basil leaves. Stir, top with a handful of ice cubes, and drink. It's so refreshing!

Spicy Green Juice

Okay, this one has a nice kick; as it includes Jalapeño that proves green juices can be really exciting and adventurous.

Ingredients:
- 1/2 Cup of Fresh Pineapple
- 5 Kale Leaves

- ½ Piece of Fresh Jalapeño
- 1 Cucumber

You could use a full jalapeño if you're feeling brave, but remember to warn your friends first!

Citrus Green Juice

If you can't handle the heat but still want a green juice that comes with a bit of a kick, try this citrus-inspired juice that proves green juicing can be tropical.

Ingredients:
- 1 Orange
- 2 Kale Leaves
- 3 Celery Stalks
- ½ Grapefruit
- ½ Cucumber
- ½ Lemon

Green Juice Cleanse

Here is one made with simple greens when you want to cleanse your body and get a big nutrition boost. This one is nice and simple and contains the classic dark leafy greens.

Ingredients:
- 4-5 Handfuls of Spinach
- 3 Kale Leaves
- 2 Green Apples
- 3 Celery Stalks
- 1 Cucumber

- ½ Lemon

Liquid Broccoli Zinger

Ingredients:
- 1 Bunch of Broccoli (Florets and Stalks)
- 2 Green Apples
- 1 Lime
- ½ Grapefruit
- 1/2 Small Zucchini
- Handful of Spinach or Romaine Lettuce Leaves
- 3 Stalks of Celery

Green Honeymoon

Ingredients:
- 1 Cucumber
- 1 Apple
- ¼ Cup of Pineapple
- 4 Kale Leaves
- 3 Swiss Chard Leaves

A Word of Caution

One pitfall is to avoid becoming so enamored with green juice that you forget about the other good stuff. You focus on kale and spinach, but you forget about beets and tomatoes. You buy lots of cabbages and broccoli, but you ignore the apples and carrots.

This is somewhat problematic because, although green vegetables are great for you, nutritionists and health experts all around the world will tell you that there is nothing better than a well-balanced diet - and this extends to a well-balanced diet of fruits and vegetables when juicing.

If you eat just certain kinds of vegetables, you'll be healthy. Sure. However, if you eat a wide variety of fruit and vegetables, you'll be even healthier.

So, get into green juicing but don't make every single juice green. Be creative and dynamic; experiment and explore a variety of colorful vegetables to add to your juice.

20 Ways to Enjoy Raw

Vegetables

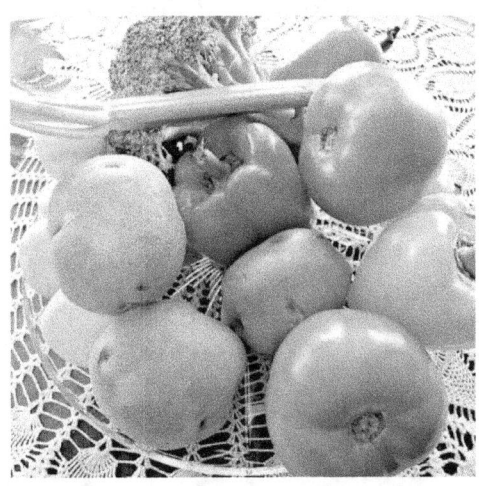

Raw Vegetables and Your Health

For some, the thought of eating vegetables is almost too much to bear, and while eating raw vegetables might not sound that appealing, there are numerous health benefits to doing so:

- Very low in calories
- No fat in the vegetables themselves and fat saved from eliminating the cooking process
- No cholesterol
- Rich in essential vitamins, minerals, enzymes and antioxidants
- Certain vegetables, like those of the cruciferous family, including, greens and broccoli are strongly

believed by scientists to have real anti-cancer
properties
- The nutrients in vegetables play a key role in
maintaining good health, including lowering risks
for heart disease, and boosting immunity
- Rich in fiber that is filling so you eat less for
healthy weight management

20 Ways to Eat and Enjoy Raw Vegetables

Raw vegetables can be enjoyed in a multitude of ways
that are not the boring, traditional variety that actually
makes them interesting to eat, follow these tips to improve
your intake of these very nutritious gems of nature.

Exciting Salads

Salad does not need to be the stereotypical salad of
dry, slightly brown lettuce leaves with a bit of tomato and
cucumber. There are never-ending possibilities when it
comes to salads, only limited by your taste buds and
imagination.

Salads don't have to be boring. You can throw in a little
cheese or grilled chicken breast. Add a wide assortment of
raw vegetables.

To make salads more interesting, combine different
color leaves, grate or finely chop some carrots, celery, red
onion, cabbage, and broccoli and combine.

Peppers, lettuce, and carrots are great choices and you
can add various herbs, like cilantro, parsley, and basil for
a little extra flavor. For variety, add in unique flavors of

herbs or spices such as mint or dill. You could even add some lemon, grapefruit, or lime juice for a tangy citrus flavor.

Grilled vegetables can be combined with raw salad fixings to make a wonderfully tasty blend. Grill some purple onions, red, green, and yellow peppers and add to a hearty lettuce like Romaine, along with cherry tomatoes, carrot slivers and raw mushroom slices, delicious!

Depending on your dietary preferences, you may wish to add beans, pulses, or lentils to the salad to make a hearty meal.

If you love the sweet/savory combination of flavors, add sweet berries to your savory salads.

The phytochemicals and vitamin C in onions boost immunity. They also contain chromium that helps to regulate blood sugar along with properties that help reduce inflammation and heal infections. A Cornell University study found that raw onions contain sulphur compounds, and cancer-fighting antioxidants that are only present in their juice. These nutrients help protect against lung and prostate cancer.

Raw onions go great with chopped cucumbers, tomatoes and dill drizzled with oil and white vinegar, a salad traditionally enjoyed in Russian cooking. Finely chopped raw sweet onion also tastes great in any type of salad as it adds a tangy sweetness and a very unique flavor that marinades well with other vegetables and various dressings.

Raw onion can also be enjoyed over any type of grilled meat, fish, or chicken.

Juicing

As juicers are so popular and affordable, it's a great idea to invest in one. You can quickly and easily juice raw produce and greatly increase your nutritional profile with an influx off fresh vitamins, minerals, enzymes, and antioxidants that are easily absorbed by the body in juice forms. If you really need to get those veggies into your body, but hate eating them, juicing is a great option.

Dips

With a food processor making a dip becomes exceptionally easy – simply throw in all the ingredients, including raw vegetables, whizz it and you're done. There are numerous options that you could make out of raw vegetables such as creamy cucumber or creamy dill. For nonfat or low fat options, swap the sour cream or mayonnaise used in dip recipes with nonfat or low-fat Greek yogurt.

You could also use carrot or celery sticks instead of breadsticks and dip them in your favorite dip.

Salsa

Salsa goes with everything, including eggs, omelets, in salads, as a dip for fresh veggies and even fruit and as a condiment in sandwiches and wraps. Fresh salsa even tastes good by itself.

You don't have to limit yourself to just tomatoes, onion, and hot peppers found in the typical salsa recipe.

You can add finely chopped raw carrot, bell peppers, celery and even chucks of raw mushrooms.

Smoothies

Smoothies are great for people on the go or who have limited time, yet still want to eat healthily. All you need is some vegetables and a blender. Throw in your favorite vegetables, with some added greens for the health benefits, such as kale or spinach, and you're done. You could add an avocado if you want a boost of healthy fat and to thicken the mixture.

Yogurt is also great in making smoothies with both raw vegetables and fruits.

Dressings

Raw vegetables, when combined with ingredients such as lemon juice and salt, make excellent dressings. These could be used on salads, meat, fish, in wraps or over grilled chicken.

Combine vegetables such as onion and garlic with apple cider vinegar or olive oil to make an excellent addition to any salad.

Snacks

Raw vegetables make excellent choices for eating on the go. It's incredibly easy to chop some cucumber, tomatoes, carrot, or peppers and pop them into a container. Within minutes, you have a healthy snack that you can eat anywhere. Combine with a dip for added flavor.

Sweet Tooth Option

Most people have a sweet tooth of some sort, and some people crave sugar much more than others. There is a way to get your sugar fix and still eat raw vegetables; some vegetables are naturally sweeter than others are so these can satisfy that craving for sugar. Choose vegetables such as squash, cherry and grape tomatoes, and carrots for healthier sweet tooth satisfaction.

Homemade Slaw

Traditional slaw often contains a large dose of mayonnaise, which is not the healthiest option. However, you can make homemade slaw taste just as good and much healthier.

Combine raw vegetables such as carrot and cabbage, and either add a small amount of low-fat or olive oil mayonnaise, or consider adding a different dressing for a more unique flavor, including Asian ginger dressings, a Greek yogurt dressing or a simple olive oil and vinegar blend.

Spiralize The Vegetables

Certain vegetable such as zucchini and carrots make excellent noodles if you have a spiralizer. If not, most peelers will give you a similar sort of effect. Once you have a handful of vegetable noodles, you can do so many things with them. You could add them to salads for extra taste and effect, or combine them with a marinara or meat sauce to make a heartier meal.

Replace Traditional Foods with Vegetables

Certain foods such as breadsticks, rice, and bread can all be replaced with raw vegetables. Lettuce or kale leaves make excellent alternatives to bread, and can be used to make a wrap or sandwich.

Cauliflower, when broken down into tiny pieces, makes an excellent alternative to rice. This can give you texture and taste in a salad or as a side dish.

Finally, vegetables such as carrots and peppers can be just as good with dips as bread.

Spice Things Up

If you find vegetables to be bland and tasteless, then you're not alone. Many people are not satisfied with a little salt and pepper so if you want to make things more interesting, just add a little spice. You can experiment with flavors, such as cumin, cayenne pepper, garlic, and even cloves.

Side Dishes

Raw vegetables make excellent side dishes at dinner. Whether it is a small salad, dips or noodle salad, all are healthy alternatives to many other traditional side dishes, especially potatoes. This is particularly the case when combined with ingredients such as cheese or fish – the possibilities are endless.

Vegetable Fondue Dippers

Who doesn't love fondue? Raw vegetables are great when dipped into a gooey, cheesy flavorful fondue and when you swap the usual bread, and meats that are dipped in fondue with raw carrots, celery, mushrooms, grape tomatoes, zucchini and even bell peppers you save a ton of calories too!

Keep Vegetables Within Easy Reach

If you fill your fridge with junk food, then you're going to eat junk food. If you have your fresh vegetables hidden away in a vegetable drawer, you'll never see them and consequently won't eat them. Preparer your veggies by washing and drying them and keeping them in clear containers at eye level in your fridge. That way, when you go to get a snack, you'll see prepared vegetables sitting in front of you.

Keep It Simple

You don't have to make a gourmet meal every time you eat. If you're spending the whole time focusing on preparation and making something that looks like a work of art, you'll see healthy food as a chore.

You should try to choose recipes that are quick and simple that you can make as quickly as you could grab a snack; this is very motivating and will make it easier for you to get your fill of healthy foods.

Involve The Whole Family

When you go shopping for food, you may find that your family's eating habits can cause you to stray from your healthy eating plan. If you want to eat more raw vegetables, you could turn the food shopping into a competition to see which family member can make the healthiest choices. This is an especially useful way to get kids involved in healthy eating and learning to make healthy choices.

Choose The Vegetables You Like

If you try to eat vegetables that you really don't like just because they're healthy, you're not going to be able to stick to your diet for long. There is no point in punishing yourself just to be healthy. If there are certain vegetables that you just can't stomach, leave them out. Just choose the vegetables you do like and enjoy and you'll find it much easier to eat veggies more often.

Add Vegetables Slowly

If you're not used to eating raw vegetables, it's probably not a good idea to replace all your usual food with raw vegetables all at once. Instead, give your taste buds and your body time to adjust to the new lifestyle by adding raw vegetables gradually to your diet. Start small and build on it.

Engage with Healthy Friends

If you join a health club, and make friends with health-minded people, you'll find that it's much easier to stick to your new routine. Eating healthy raw vegetables with other people will encourage you to make healthier choices and you won't feel like you're missing out as you might watch friends eat junk food.

Conclusion

Your body needs the micronutrients found in fruit and vegetables, 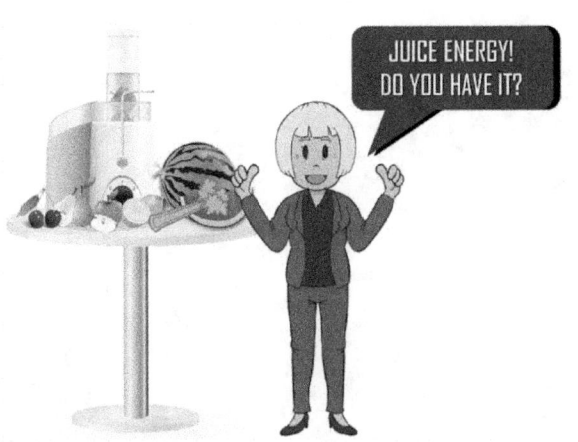 and juicing is a really great way of getting them. Furthermore, if you don't enjoy eating whole produce, juicing can help you get key nutrients that vegetables provide.

In fact, one large glass of juice is like eating 2 large salads without the fattening dressing.

You don't have to juice every single day, but it's great if you can make it a fundamental part of your daily routine.

Because most people who start juicing tend to really love it, it invariably becomes a crucial part of their daily routine. It becomes a habit that they don't ever want to lose.

There are just so many benefits...

You feel more energized

More alert

Your immune system gets a boost

Your bones are strengthened

You stay hydrated

Your skin looks better

You supply your body with the nutrition it needs to fight disease

And you may lose some weight...

What More Could You Ask for?

ABOUT THE AUTHOR

Rod is an author, publisher, consultant, and provider of information on health, nutrition and work from home in order to improve your life.

Rod is the principle partner of **Rod Stone Group** and their main company **r Healthy Living Solutions** focus on providing information on health, nutrition, and work from home in order to improve your life. With over two dozen experts providing content, they are able to provide some of the most useful information you will find.

Rod began writing articles on health and nutrition in the mid '90s. In 2004 he started full time working with people and providing information and products to assist with health and nutrition. In 2008 he started to become involved with the importance of specialized high intensity workouts.

We have also started to provide products on Amazon and information can be found at their main information site http://rhealthylivingsolutions.com. At here you can get access to the articles that are posted daily and join the **Free book a month club. With the book a month club we will send you a monthly e-book on healthy living and personal development topics.**

The other books in the Healthy Food Series which are all available on Amazon are:

Health Tips: Over 500 tips for your health

Vegetables*: Learn to Enjoy More Varieties While Benefitting Your Health*

Vegetable recipes from the past*: Learn how to enjoy vegetables for your health*

Nutrients for Health*: Your guide to foods and nutrients for your health and for overcoming ailments*

Salads for any occasion*: Salads can be much more than just a side dish*

Learning to Eat Healthy*: Find out what your body needs and how to shop; store; and prepare for the best in taste and health*

Improve your life,

Rod

www.ingramcontent.com/pod-product-compliance
Lightning Source LLC
Chambersburg PA
CBHW062139280526
45788CB00001B/229